Food Microbiology and Food Safety
Practical Approaches

Series Editor
Michael P. Doyle

T0186010

Food Microbiology and Food Safety: Practical Approaches

The Food Microbiology and Food Safety series is published in conjunction with the International Association for Food Protection, a non-profit association for food safety professionals. Dedicated to the life-long educational needs of its Members, IAFP provides an information network through its two scientific journals (Food Protection Trends and Journal of Food Protection), its educational Annual Meeting, international meetings and symposia, and interaction between food safety professionals.

Series Editor

Michael P. Doyle, *Regents Professor and Director of the Center for Food Safety, University of Georgia, Griffith, GA, USA*

Editorial Board

For further volumes:
http://www.springer.com/series/11567

Hal King

Food Safety Management

Implementing a Food Safety Program
in a Food Retail Business

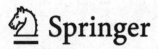 Springer

Hal King, Ph.D.
110 Parliament Ct.
Fayetteville, GA, USA

ISBN 978-1-4939-0199-9   ISBN 978-1-4614-6205-7 (eBook)
DOI 10.1007/978-1-4614-6205-7
Springer New York Heidelberg Dordrecht London

Printed on acid-free paper

Springer is part of Springer Science+Business Media (www.springer.com)

This book is dedicated to my lovely wife, Karen Lynn King, for all the love and support she has provided me to enhance my work all these years. To KK, my wife, my love, and my best friend!

Foreword

Passion for what you do is often the key to success. When Hal King asked me to write the foreword to this book, I gladly accepted. Having worked in the food safety, technical, operations, and business areas of the food industry (from farm to fork) myself for over 35 years, I recognized the need for a book that provides both current and future food safety professionals with guidelines on how to effectively do their jobs. Hal has a passion for food safety. I have worked with him professionally and watched him not only develop programs but also successfully implement them. This book also draws on Hal's experience as a public health professional.

Food safety is a moral imperative. Getting others to implement, maintain, and continuously improve a food safety management program that leads to the prevention of foodborne illnesses is a challenge that requires persuasion and diligence. Hal has addressed this very effectively. He shows how to communicate the food safety management program's value so that those who use them understand their importance and also how they will have a positive effect on many of the areas in which they are assessed. The need and value of a food safety management program must be communicated in a manner to which the C-level (CEO, COO, CFO, VP of Operations, VP of Purchasing) and other influencers and users of the information can relate. Management commitment, as discussed, is required for the success of the food safety management program and for the food safety professionals to get the resources they need. These resources include the people, money, and departmental cooperation needed to effectively implement the components of the food safety management program.

One of the things often lacking in the food safety professional's education and experience is an understanding of the business areas within their company. Without this understanding, the food safety professional cannot effectively communicate with others or develop metrics that demonstrate the value of having an effective food safety management program. This book highlights this need and suggests ways to gain this knowledge.

Hal identifies and discusses the various types of food safety management program components along with the education (why) and training (how) needed to implement these programs. Particular emphasis is paid to the need to educate. Experience has shown that explaining why something needs to be done and then applying the rules helps the responsible individual to more effectively do their job. To emphasize this, I remember sitting in a lecture many years ago in which the speaker demonstrated the need for education along with training. He asked the audience who among them could name the Ten Commandments. The only one in the group who said they could name all ten was a theologian. We have probably heard all ten often and for the most part have been educated as to their meaning. But to name all ten was difficult. With this in mind, ask yourself if you really expect a person to remember a great number of food safety rules without the benefit of the underlying food safety education.

Other important areas to understand in effectively implementing a food safety management program are interrelations with other departments. Hal discusses how to work with key areas such as product development, R&D, purchasing, engineering, equipment design, sanitation, and maintenance groups. As a first step in planning the food safety management program, you must understand what you need within your organization and what is already in place. This becomes the basis for your planning and implementation activities. By using the Gap analysis protocol which Hal describes, you will be able to get an accurate picture of the situation. By combining this with a review of best industry practices, the most effective food safety management program can be developed.

Of particular interest is how Hal uses his experience as a public health official throughout this book and to explain the value of working with this important resource and how to effectively do so. Above all, this is a hands-on guidebook that can be used to develop and implement an effective food safety management program. It is written by a well-recognized expert in the industry who provides both the dos and don'ts. Both current and future food safety professionals will benefit from this book.

Gary Ades, Ph.D.

Acknowledgments

First, I have to thank Mr. S. Truett Cathy for taking time away from his work to teach me the value of work, the importance of character and making good decisions, and doing business with a focus on helping others succeed. After knowing him first for over 30 years as a friend and trusted councilor, I currently work for the company he created applying these principles. Second, I need to thank my former doctoral thesis professor, Dr. Emmett Shotts Jr. (University of Georgia School of Veterinary Medicine), who encouraged me to discover and challenged me to be my best. He introduced me to and guided me through the detailed science of public health, leading me to work at the Centers for Disease Control and Prevention. I would like to thank Dr. Tom Shinnick and Dr. Barry Fields (at CDC), both of whom supported all my ideas and allowed me the freedom to learn investigative principles and the science of infectious disease epidemic investigations. I would like to thank Dr. David Stephens (Emory University School of Medicine) for giving me the amazing opportunity to lead an academic laboratory built to investigate infectious diseases, which allowed me the honor, in some small way, to build upon the knowledge base to prevent them. Finally, I must thank my current boss and friend, Mr. Tom Childers. Although the content of this book comes from my own experience working to build a food safety management program, very little of it would have taken form without his trusted guidance and counsel (and patience with a public health professional that wanted everything done now) in the business of food safety.

Contents

Chapter 1
Introduction

Before you read this book, first let me tell you about who is writing it and why. I first became interested in writing this book a year after I started my first industry-related job where I became responsible for leading food and product safety at a major food retail business. Prior to this job, I had extensive training and experience in management as a government chief scientist in the US Public Health Service (at the Centers for Disease Control and Prevention, Epidemic Investigations Laboratories), as a military biological threats officer (United States Army Reserves, Consequence Management Unit), and as a university assistant research professor (Infectious Diseases Division of Emory University School of Medicine). However, I had little business experience nor could I find a specific resource on how to lead a retail organizations food safety management program.

The food retail business I work for is a restaurant company that buys ingredients, products, and packaging, from various manufactures; distributes these components to currently over 1,700 plus restaurants in 39 states and District of Columbia; and then produces/packages fresh made food in these restaurants, serving over two million customers a day. When I became the one responsible for food and product safety within this organization (literally concerned about the public health of over two million customers a day), I started to look at this responsibility first as a public health professional, studying the risk, requesting resources, and developing and implementing tools and procedures as a means for the intervention of the risk. I quickly learned, though, that this was only part of the process. I needed to learn how to integrate this public health scope into the business processes within the organization if I was to be successful in sustaining the benefits of my professional input.

So I did what most business professionals already do; I built relationships with key stakeholders within my organization to learn their business needs, studied the management methods of other food safety professionals within the food industry, sought knowledge through public health organizations tasked to regulate food safety, and studied peer-reviewed publications and books. I also traveled to attend national food safety organizational meetings (e.g., Food Safety Summit, International Association for Food Protection, National Environmental Health Association,

H. King, *Food Safety Management: Implementing a Food Safety Program in a Food Retail Business*, Food Microbiology and Food Safety, DOI 10.1007/978-1-4614-6205-7_1,
© Springer Science+Business Media New York 2013

American Society of Microbiology) and took courses in public health management developed by Harvard School of Public Health and risk management training at the FDA's Joint Institute for Food Safety and Nutrition (JIFSAN). Through this journey, I developed the knowledge to build a model that helped me organize and manage the work necessary to ensure food safety in a food retail business. You may be wondering why I didn't ask other food safety business professionals to write different chapters of this book or provide their management principals as part of my thesis. This certainly could have expanded the scope with different perspectives used to successfully manage food safety in a retail organization; perhaps a book with these perspectives should be written next. However, my primary objective was to write this book from the perspective of a public health professional that has researched, bench marked, and applied many of the best practices in food safety directly to the management of a retail food safety management program. The reader can fill in additional knowledge as it relates to the specific needs/culture of their retail food business using this book as a guide.

Public Health Responsibility

Many food safety professionals who have worked and currently work in the food retail industry work with the same dedication and initiative as most public health professionals tasked to prevent foodborne illnesses; just look at the names on the boards and membership list of most industry trade and nonprofit originations that support food safety improvement (including professional development groups within these organizations). Each of these food safety professionals take on the difficult responsibility for food safety within their organization (i.e., are held accountable for food safety), and also many work outside of their organizations to foster improvements in retail food safety (via benchmarking, service on local, state, and federal government boards, speaking/training, writing, etc.) seeing food safety as a noncompetitive part of the business.

Even though public health (CDC, FDA, USDA), academic scientist, and retail and manufacturing food safety professionals have worked together for many years to improve food safety, we continue to see unnecessary outbreaks of foodborne illnesses and deaths similar to the tragic events of the past that initiated public demand to improve. Take, for example, the multistate outbreak of listeriosis linked to whole cantaloupes from Jensen Farms in Colorado, United States, in 2011. Without going into the details of how this outbreak occurred (some of which is still speculative), cantaloupes were linked to 147 illnesses and 33 deaths (and one miscarriage due to the illness) in 28 states (CDC 2012a). Unfortunately, based on our current means to communicate national recalls of adulterated foods (via press reports by the government and/or industry), and poor means to quickly trace back foods to original sources of cultivation and/or production, the outbreak continued to cause illnesses and deaths 47 days (see Fig. 1.1) after the announcement of the likely source of the outbreak (whole or fresh cut cantaloupes linked to Jensen Farms).

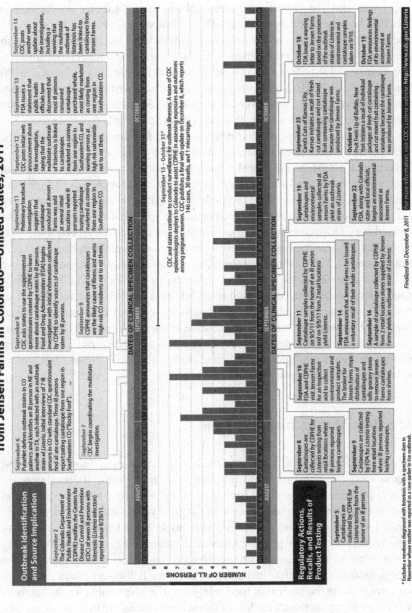

Fig. 1.1 Epidemiological timeline of illnesses caused by cantaloupes showing numbers of persons who became ill even after the FDA recall was announced on September 13, 2011 (CDC 2012a)

According to Flynn (2012), Jensen Farms has filed bankruptcy and is part of a criminal investigation by the state of Colorado, and the outbreak has resulted in civil legal actions by most of the victims or their survivors. A third party auditing firm used by Jensen farms, Texas-based Bio Food Safety, also filed bankruptcy.

Over a year after the outbreak, the estimated cost of medical care was $8 million (expected to be more in future medical bills and lost wages) for only 42 of the 147 sick persons the CDC was able to indentify (more were likely), and the cost to industry (including retail food businesses that sold these cantaloupes), government, and the families (due to lost loved ones/lost wages) is estimated to be over $100 million (Marler 2012). Most interesting is that as I sit here writing this book, another outbreak has been reported with over 141 illnesses in 20 states, 31 hospitalized, and two deaths, from cantaloupes again, this time due to *Salmonella typhimurium* (CDC 2012b). Clearly we need to get better if we are going to change this, and it must be regulatory/investigative agencies and industry working together.

Government public health (local, state, and federal) agencies are tasked to research (along with academic partners funded by these agencies), design, and implement regulatory requirements to protect the public health. The government oftentimes provides the means for industry to provide input on the feasibility of these regulatory requirements to help ensure they are cost effective, but some food safety regulatory requirements will cost more money to implement (expected cost of doing business). The food retail business has a responsibility to partner with these public health agencies in the prevention of foodborne illnesses. More importantly, the food safety professionals in a food retail business can influence food safety as buyers of manufactured foods for its retail units by requiring and verifying manufacturers are following the most current science to prevent food safety hazards during food production. This responsibility is equal to specifying and verifying that their own retail units are following the most current science to prevent food safety hazards during retail food production.

Food Safety Management Program

It is my desire that this book will provide you with the basics of "how to" lead and manage a food safety management program in your business. It contains many examples of successful programs I have used in my retail food business career and knowledge I acquired through working with the great people where I work presently to ensure food safety for our customers. This book is written for the food safety business professional with a primary focus on the managers responsible for leading and supervising (or those tasked with organizing a food safety management team) a retail organization's food safety management program. It also serves as a significant resource for training the student of food safety (anyone responsible for the safety of our food must always remain a student of this science) including the student seeking a degree in food science/safety or the business student/professional tasked to learn how to manage people and work within a retail organization that requires a food safety program.

It is my hope that when you have read this book, you will have learned:

- How to develop and lead a food safety management program/department from a national brand perspective
- Provide the proper organization to manage the work necessary to ensure food safety is a priority within all business functions in the organization (from supplier to retail units)
- Provide the systems, broad specifications, and expected training/education and facility design needs to manage food safety risk in each business function
- Demonstrate examples that can be used for continuous improvement in sustaining and building upon the food safety benefits achieved by the food safety management program
- Provide methods to gain influence and obtain resources to support food safety responsibilities within the business
- Develop important relationships with public health professionals based on new science and current regulatory compliance to ensure cost effective business management

How to Use This Book

This book is organized into chapters based on the foundational core components of a food safety management program necessary to achieve maximum value of the investment you make in people and programs within your organization. Several of these components have dual function/overlap in other departments in the business including the company's supply chain, distribution system, business analysis, marketing, faculties management/real estate, and its retail point of sales operations. The critical component of a food safety management program is *commitment* (Fig. 1.2). Chapter 2 will focus on the implementation of commitment which is the selection of the right people to manage food safety responsibilities (the food safety management team) to ensure successful program management and continuous improvement. This discussion is purposely first because if this is not introduced into the organization as part of its DNA, then all the other recommendations in subsequent chapters will likely not be sustainable. The right people are then empowered to lead a food safety management program and influence other departments through leadership of defined core responsibilities with the program (Chap. 3). Each team manager owns responsibilities of the three primary business functions (retail units, supplier manufacturing facilities, and regulatory compliance), and is enabled to identify and develop methods to reduce risk (Fig. 1.2) in each.

The next four chapters discuss the core components (see Fig. 1.2) of the food safety management program responsibilities (systems, training and education, facilities and capabilities, and execution and verification). In Chap. 4, systems are defined and how the food safety team uses them to control and prevent food safety hazards across all the business functions of the organization. This includes the authority of the team to influence decisions on who the organization partners with (reviewed

Fig. 1.2 Organization of a food safety management program's components, the business function areas that manage these components, and the continuous improvement process via Gap analysis

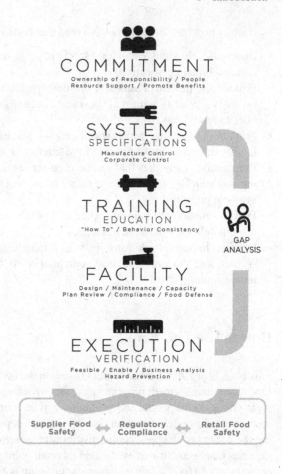

annually) to produce its food in the supply chain and retail outlets. In education and training (Chap. 5) and facilities and capabilities (Chap. 6), the necessary processes to enable all the food safety specifications are discussed. To enable a true program management process, execution and verification of each of the individual core components of the program are measured (Chap. 7). This is also necessary to identify areas needed to improve compliance and ensure a continuous food safety focus within the business. Another function of the food safety management program is the management of a third party gap analysis (Chap. 8) of the food retail business to identify gaps within the business that may need to be filled with new systems, training and education, or facilities design improvements; this includes a process to repeat the gap analysis on a regular basis (based on risk) to ensure no new gaps within the food safety management program and the business functions develop over time (Fig. 1.2). Although resources must be in place to initiate the work on the core components described, commitment is sustained by a process the food safety management team uses to gain the resources within the organization necessary to improve and then sustain the investment in food safety (Chap. 9). In other words, the food safety management team must be able to show value via the business analysis process to compete for organizational dollars each year.

Compliance to the continually changing regulatory environment is discussed through the lenses of partnerships with public health officials (Chap. 10). Current well-defined regulatory requirements will naturally form the basis of all specifications and systems as discussed in Chap. 4. However, Chap. 10 is separate from the foundational core components of the food safety management program because regulatory actions can increase the cost of doing business (reducing profit), and well-formed partnerships based on documented regulatory compliance are necessary, and may reduce the cost to the retail organization by leveraging mutually desired public health goals to reduce food safety risk in the supply chain. The *references* in the back of each chapter are mostly "how to" sources and heavy on citing internet web sites to aid the reader in using additional resources immediately for food safety management program development.

I encourage you to use this book as a guide for applying your own more specific details that you develop within your organization's culture and business model to ensure success. Because the science of food safety is always improving due to the work of food safety professionals in government, academia, and industry, this book can't possibly cover all aspects of food safety management, nor all the systems and other solutions to reduce the risk of a foodborne illness within the retail food business. You must remain a student of the many excellent resources (peer-reviewed journals, books, and trade articles) written by experts in all areas of food safety science and several national and international organizations that support the development and communication of this science, including the publishers of this book.

Ultimately, the responsibility of food safety within an organization comes down to people (which is the focus of the next chapter of this book) and their desire (and the organization's commitment to empower them) to "own" the responsibility of food safety. The prevention of human suffering that can result from a foodborne illness makes food safety a public health responsibility and necessary function of the food retail business. Second to this, the negative impact of any foodborne illness on the company's brand should motivate all decisions by a retail food business. The right people, carefully managing the risk in collaboration with other business and regulatory professionals within and outside the organization, are the best means to ensure food safety within the food retail business.

Finally, this book is intended to start the dialog on how to best develop and maintain a food safety management program in a food retail business. It is my hope that other experienced food safety professionals will continue this dialog via publication of effective methods within their programs to help us all succeed in this public health responsibility. If you, as a food safety professional would like to provide feedback and additional ideas/improvements on how a retail food business can manage food safety in support of its public health responsibilities, I welcome these on my blog, Public Health Responsibilities of a Food Retail Business at http://publichealthresponsibilitie-sofafoodrb.blogspot.com/. I will try to use these inputs and additional research to improve this book in subsequent editions.

References

CDC (2012a) Multistate outbreak of Listeriosis linked to whole cantaloupes from Jensen Farms, Colorado. Centers for Disease Control and Prevention Outbreak Highlights. Available via internet at http://www.cdc.gov/listeria/outbreaks/cantaloupes-jensen-farms/index.html

CDC (2012b) Multistate outbreak of *Salmonella* Typhimurium infections linked to cantaloupe. Available via internet at http://www.cdc.gov/salmonella/typhimurium-cantaloupe-08-12/index.html

Flynn D (2012) Deadly *Listeria* Outbreak Focus of Federal Criminal Probe. Food Safety News. Available via internet at http://www.foodsafetynews.com/2012/08/deadly-listeria-outbreak-focus-of-criminal-probe/?utm_source=newsletter&utm_medium=email&utm_campaign=120815

Marler B (2012) Publisher's platform: ode to the microbiological data program. Food Safety News. Available via internet at http://www.foodsafetynews.com/2012/08/publishers-platform-ode-to-microbiological-data-program/

Chapter 2
The Food Safety Management Team

> *Own: to have or hold as property; to have power or mastery over; to acknowledge to be true, valid, or as claimed*

Merriam Webster 2012

Having people in the food safety management program empowered to own the responsibility to reduce risk within a retail food business is an important factor in the organizations success to prevent foodborne diseases. This alone is a significant means to measure the commitment of the food retail business to food safety. Each individual food safety management team member continuously works to understand risk, initiates new projects to reduce risk, and is the leader in protecting the brand through vigilant surveillance of risk. Selection of the mangers on this team is critical to the success of the program. The team members must be trained in the business of public health (subject matter experts on the prevention strategies to prevent a foodborne disease) and know how to work within cross-functional teams within the core functions of the business including the supplier food safety, regulatory compliance, and retail food safety functions.

Empowered to Own Responsibility

A restaurant owner, we'll call her Sara, noticed that every time the local health inspector visited her restaurant, she was always cited for poor sanitation. The water they stored the cloth towels in was never at the right concentration of sanitizer strength (food code requires that reused cloth towels be kept in the appropriate strength of sanitizer to ensure the towels don't spread germs). She and her employees knew this requirement well, and they always kept the kitchen looking clean (she was at the restaurant most of the time helping fill orders or cleaning between food prep). However, she also knew it was next to impossible to maintain the proper level of sanitizer in a pail of water when the same towel was used over and over to wipe up food debris, oil, grease, and raw foods.

H. King, *Food Safety Management: Implementing a Food Safety Program in a Food Retail Business*, Food Microbiology and Food Safety, DOI 10.1007/978-1-4614-6205-7_2,
© Springer Science+Business Media New York 2013

"Using towels stored in buckets of water was the way restaurants always did this wasn't it, and why was her restaurant being singled out all the time when this was the way health departments wanted cloth towels used." She tried to require her employees to change the water every few hours, increase the strength of the sanitizer at the beginning of the day, made check list to try and reinforce proper use, and yet she still got "dinged" by the health inspector; it was just next to impossible to do. Reusing cloth towels to clean surfaces reminded her of when customers use to reuse the same unsanitary cloth towel to dry hands; "remember those rotating cloth towel dispensers they use to have in gas station restrooms." That industry got rid of those towels didn't they, and now they use disposable paper towels or blow dryers? Sara knew the inspector was correct in enforcing this rule, "he was just doing his job," but couldn't someone come up with a more operationally feasible method?

So Sara decided to investigate other methods to clean and sanitize surfaces without using a dirty reused towel stored in a pail of water. After all, she wouldn't clean this way in her own kitchen at home, so why did she do this in her restaurant where she serves a great deal more people. The obvious solution was disposable wipes that already had the proper sanitizer strength built into the wipe and a means to dispense the wipes so that employees would use them properly when they cleaned and sanitized surfaces. Germs would be thrown away each time they cleaned and no more dirty bucket of water and lower health department scores. All Sara had to do was find someone to make them; this would be a game changer, and she could also save on laundry of cloth towels as well. Sara found a company that made disposable wipes and asked them to make a new dispenser to look like the red sanitizer buckets all restaurants used (but only to dispense disposable sanitizer wipes). Her employees loved the new system, the health inspector was impressed with how the employees now "toss out the germs," and Sara was confident her restaurant had the cleanest and safest kitchen in town. Using her business savvy (knowing cost would likely prohibit use of a disposable wipe compared to reusing cloth towels), Sara developed a recycling program with the manufacturer to make their use cost neutral with laundry, chemical, and labor cost of maintaining reused cloth towels.

The most important asset a food retail business can have leading its food safety management program is the right people in the right position empowered with the responsibility of food safety for their customers like they are the owners of the business. People who have a stake in something tend to take more responsibility for it like Sara the restaurant owner in the previous story. These people challenge the status quo when things are not working as they should, desire change when improvement is needed, measure their impact continually, and ultimately improve the outcome of the business simply because they desire continuous improvement. These people also empower others in continuous improvement knowing that more rapid change comes from more people working who are aligned to the change.

People who are empowered to own responsibility like Sara in this story oftentimes also act expectantly for the general good of the public. In this case, Sara created an easier means to clean and sanitize food contact surfaces in a retail food establishment that others can use to reduce food safety risk in their restaurants as well. James Q. Wilson, a noted Harvard Professor and political scientist, stated (speaking about what motivates people to do the right thing in their business without a need for regulatory oversight), "perhaps the most powerful antidote to unfettered selfishness is property rights. .... If we are catching lobsters off the Maine coast, we can restrict over-fishing by allocating spaces to groups who informally "own" each space" (Wall Street 2012). The business people in Dr. Wilson's example likely already protect natural resources necessary to sustain their business through ownership, but they are much more likely to do so if they are empowered to work as if they own it. All food retail businesses can benefit through this same type of ownership, in this case, to prevent foodborne illnesses, by treating the business of food safety as a noncompetitive responsibility.

Selecting the Food Safety Management Team

So, how do you find the right people that you can trust to empower with this food safety ownership? First and foremost, they must have demonstrated competency and integrity in their previous work and have demonstrated this competency in reducing risk for another organization. In my current business culture, we describe this as the three C's for character, competency, and chemistry which was first introduced as a template to hire great leaders by Bill Hybels in his book Courageous Leadership (Hybels 2002). Mr. Truett Cathy, the founder and CEO of Chick-fil-A, has said in many of his interviews and books, and I am paraphrasing this, "that you can train for competency if you have to, but it's difficult to create character; look for character first then competency and chemistry".

Of course competency is a requirement for a food safety management team member, but without character, the competency may be misdirected and not focused on the public health of the organizations customers. There's an old saying that you don't find buzzards where eagles fly, so if you want an eagle, go to where they fly. The best places to find competent food safety professionals with character are places where people are demonstrating success in promoting the science of public health. These professionals are already seeking to know more about food safety risk and how to mitigate this risk for their current organization. For example, graduate students who are pursuing an advanced science or public health degree undergo rigorous critical scrutiny of their work, must often initiate and prove new ideas, and manage projects to completion, and errors are rarely tolerated for advancement of their thesis. Thus, graduate schools of public health and food science are the first places to look to find food safety management team members.

Let me tell you a story that teaches an important lesson on the evidence that you have selected the right people to own their job responsibilities. This story is about me (so its firsthand experience), but I was only the student (and employee) being taught by someone of great character and competency, and it taught me responsibility, but also how to look for this in others before we hire them to own responsibility within our own organization. A much abbreviated part of this story was published by Mr. Truett Cathy to teach a lesson on the recipe for being happy and successful in your work in his first book, "It's Easier To Succeed Than Fail" (the book is out of print, but can still be found on the internet and used book stores). When I was working at a Chick-fil-A restaurant as an early teen, I was hoping to work the cash register or cook the food because these jobs seemed more important and fun. However, when I reported to work the first week, they wanted me to be the one that cleaned the equipment and restaurant, and I was very discouraged. Now this was an expected reaction of a 16 year old (I felt I was more qualified for other jobs, i.e., cleaning was below me and I didn't like to do it at home or work). Because I knew the founder of Chick-fil-A, Mr. Truett Cathy, I spoke with him occasionally, and he asked me how I liked the job at the restaurant.

When I told Mr. Cathy how discouraged I was, he suggested that if I wanted to be successful at work (translated: given the important jobs because I demonstrated ownership of the small ones), I should ask to clean the restrooms and then clean the toilets like I was going to drink out of them. Well, needless to say, it challenged me, but I gave it a try. I cleaned those restrooms so much that customers were afraid to go into them because I hovered over them like a hawk to keep them clean. Thus, when I approached the job like I was responsible for an important part of the business (we all know that clean restrooms are important to customers in a restaurant environment), I felt pride in my work (the founder said it was important), and the more direct benefit was the restaurant owner noticed and gave me more important duties to contribute to the success of the business. I also then knew how important that job was to the business, and even though it wasn't my job anymore, I continued to look at those restrooms to ensure they were being cleaned.

Let me tell you another story about looking for competency in those who demonstrate ownership of responsibility. I was President of the Georgia Association for Food Protection (an affiliate of the International Association for Food Protection, IAFP) during one year so I could develop relationships with other food safety and regulatory professionals. This organization had a strong program for professional development to support students and others early in their food safety careers; several students from local colleges and universities often attended these meetings. I happened to meet a fellow working on his Ph.D. who had a dream of 1 day leading my organizations' food safety department. This fellow had already demonstrated competency in his area of research on the reduction of human pathogens from raw poultry (not to mention the necessary skills to achieve a Ph.D. while working a full time job at the USDA). When I needed to find a person to lead development of food safety specifications for suppliers in my organization, the first place I looked was at who was attending these meetings and who was hungry for making things better. This fellow ultimately was recruited and now contributes significantly to the management of food safety hazards within our organization.

Although there should be no bias toward selection of graduate level professionals like Ph.D.s, these type of students have strong evidence of character and competency and provide a template for the type of person needed to manage a business function within the food safety management program. Those who obtain an advanced degree (master's or Ph.D.) have to go through a great deal of advanced education and independent project work, developing and communicating new knowledge in their respective subject matter. They must then rigorously defend their work on this new knowledge as well as demonstrate its context with current knowledge to expert peers within their field (those already with advanced degrees and experience) before they are awarded the degree.

I have also found several great people already working in different areas of the food safety profession that do not have advanced degrees but work as if they are seeking one (as evidenced by their actions), studying the issues and developing solutions to them (even on their own time). These types of professionals provide another template for selection of the types of people you need to manage food safety. One of the best responses I received from a former health inspector during an interview for a new regulatory compliance staff position in my organization, when asked why she wanted to leave her current position, was (paraphrased for emphasis) "I would like to help restaurants achieve food safety rather than just measure them for regulatory compliance." This answer was not based on what she wanted to leave but more on what she wanted to do to help retail organizations improve public health. These types of people don't need to be assigned task but rather enabled to do what they do best to reduce hazards and develop the projects necessary for continuous improvement within the organization.

Ultimately, the best way to measure if you have selected the right person that will take ownership of their individual food safety responsibilities is to see it in action. Say a manager was responsible for monitoring serous food safety issues in your supply chain (e.g., investigating the validity of calls with a supplier after a customer calls and claims they are sick from eating one of your products) and received this call while on vacation over the weekend. However, this manager did not transfer this responsibility to someone else (equally capable) or ignored the call and waited to respond until they returned to work. This manager did not demonstrate ownership of this responsibility, and the results of this one decision could be devastating to the business IF the product (and there is likely a large volume of this product in the system) was contaminated. Not only could other customers be injured, but the responsibility for initiating a recall of this product (i.e., removing it from retail service/sale) could be required by law, and this one error could cost the business significantly. Of course, this expectation should be made clear for whomever holds this level of responsibility, and everyone needs time away from work (and this type of responsibility). The point is that "owners" arc people who very rarely will allow food safety risk that may harm customers go unchecked even if they are on vacation or away from the office.

A Successful Food Safety Management Team

It would be much healthier for a business to bring food safety professionals into the organization in the beginning rather than wait for a food safety problem to occur and then look for these types of people. After a horrible series of events in 1992 that lead to the death of four children and sickened over 700 due to a common source of *Eschericia coli* 0157 infection in ground beef, the Jack in the Box chain hired a new food safety leader, Dr. Dave Theno. Dr. Theno was already working to reduce the risk of *E. coli* 0157 infections from beef as a private consultant to the National Cattleman's Beef Association. While his work ultimately improved food safety at Jack in the Box, leading the organization to win the industry coveted IAFP Black Pearl Award for Food Safety excellence, his leadership and the influence his retail food business had as a major buyer of raw red meat contributed to the improvement of food safety within the beef industry (Benedict 2011).

Finally, never delegate a food safety responsibility to a food safety management professional without providing the resources to manage this responsibility including enabling their continuous education on their specific subject matter. Once you have the right people on the food safety management team, you should enable them to measure hazards, work on continuous education and career advancement (outside your organization and among their peers to enable more ideas to prevent hazards cost effectively), and ensure they are provided the resources necessary to apply this knowledge to your organization's needs. A public health professional desires to communicate their work (i.e., as part of their professional responsibilities to share methods to prevent foodborne illnesses), teach others how to reduce risk, and work together with other food safety professionals to develop new tools of intervention that can reduce risk. Thus, the food safety professionals you select for the food safety management team will desire the same within your organization; let them. You then have influencers (see Chap. 9) in your organization that will help you integrate the teams work within the business to ensure food safety and brand protection.

References

Benedict J (2011) Poisoned. Inspired Books, Buena Vista, VA
Hybels B (2002) Courageous leadership. Zondervan, Grand Rapids, MI
Wall Street J (2012) James Q. Wilson in his own words, March 2.

Chapter 3
The Food Safety Management Program

The food safety management program focused on the identification of hazards and management of these hazards in all business functions is the most important means to ensure food safety within a food retail business. The team that manages this work within the program should be the key subject matter experts in making decisions based on factual knowledge of the food safety hazards within all business functions of the organization. Commitment to the program must be defined and supported by the organization to enable the team to effectively "study" the business and ensure systems are in place and specifications are being followed to reduce risk. When organized properly, the food safety management program adds value to the organization by preventing unnecessary cost and can even provide important evidence in the defense against false legal claims.

Commitment to a Food Safety Management Program

Commitment of the organization is the starting point of a food safety management program (see Fig. 1.2, Chap. 1). The responsibility for commitment belongs to senior leadership who must support and endorse the teams work and their influence throughout the organization. Food safety must be its priority, and this priority should be defined in a written food safety policy statement that outlines the structure and responsibilities of the food safety management program. This policy should define compliance to regulatory requirements, expectations of leadership in other departments, commitment to continuously improve the management program, and should be communicated to all employees of the organization as further evidence of the organizations food safety commitment. In addition, this policy should demonstrate:

1. A food safety expert appointed in the position of authority to lead the food safety management program.
2. Providing adequate resources (people and money) to support all elements of the food safety management program.

H. King, *Food Safety Management: Implementing a Food Safety Program in a Food Retail Business*, Food Microbiology and Food Safety, DOI 10.1007/978-1-4614-6205-7_3, © Springer Science+Business Media New York 2013

3. Set food safety educational requirements of the organization (staff outside the food safety management program) to ensure alignment of the shared responsibility for food safety in all other departments:

   - All related job descriptions must include a responsibility for food safety in each respective operational role within the business.
   - A training plan should be in place for all operational positions.

4. Creation of a food safety manual for both retail and supply chain functions of the food safety management program that includes:

   - Written procedures/requirements based on HACCP principals that identify hazards and systems and specifications as prevention controls.
   - Prerequisite programs and supporting documentation to support the policy statement on food safety for each of the business functions of the organization.

5. Communication and empowerment of responsibility to all stakeholders to report food safety issues to senior management and the food safety management team:

   - Enable method to report issues to the food safety management team.
   - Enable means to investigate and resolve/document.

6. Procedures for handling and investigating customer complaints prioritized based on risk should be documented including changes made due to complaint/claim:

   - Communicated to customers in timely manner.

7. Assurance of the execution and then verification of all food safety systems annually by senior management and when any major changes to the organization are made:

   - Support routine verification of specifications in both supply and retail business functions.
   - Changes in the food safety management program (due to discovery) must be validated, and records of all research that lead to change should be maintained.

8. A commitment to identify gaps within the food safety management program and business:

   - Performed by expert third party review.
   - Benchmarked against regulatory requirements (e.g., FDA Food Code) and industry standards (e.g., Global Food Safety Initiative, (GFSI)).

One of the best resources for how to build and measure commitment to food safety in a food business is Frank Yiannas's book on *Food Safety Culture* (Yiannas 2009). This reference is the only one currently that teaches how to create a behavior-based (i.e., ownership of responsibilities for food safety) food safety management culture and includes the specific systems and expectations of people to ensure food safety commitment within the organization. Food Safety Culture is an excellent "how to" reference for the foundation of ensuring commitment and performance of the food safety management program within your food retail organization.

Organizational Structure of the Food Safety Management Program

Before we discuss the functions of the food safety management program, we must first define the organization of the program. Several retail food organizations combine their food safety functions within a quality control/improvement department. This is likely because quality improvements have more direct correlation to daily sales and cost to the business and thus foster more internal resources for support. Many quality specifications also have dual impact with food safety benefits (e.g., temperature of food maintenance systems), and it would appear to be cost effective to have the quality team perform food safety duties. However, it is easier to identify risk, develop and resource systems and specifications to reduce them, and measure success of these systems if there is an independent food safety team focused just on food safety program management (especially if the organization is large). This team is then free to design all phases of the business's food safety needs and focus its independent resources to sustain the investment made to the business. Even if all known risks were controlled, business growth (e.g., volume) and development (e.g., new products, change in suppliers) will always require the subject matter expertise and direct focus of a food safety management program to ensure new risks are identified and controlled. These subject matter experts working together with the knowledge of all systems and requirements also serve as the "go to" persons when the need arises for product safety decisions in all areas of the business. This includes determination of operational feasibility of procedures and recipes, product development/new equipment/facilities design review to ensure food safety, and support to the business when challenges are made to the regulatory compliance of retail procedures. Most importantly, this team supports important business decisions in the event of crisis like product recalls or foodborne illness claims (legal and/or when claims are made in the media).

An important aspect of the food safety management program will be where in the organization the program is positioned and whom does it report to (i.e., its independence to provide "third party" like council). From my experience, the best place for the food safety management program is as an autonomous team/department that reports directly to the COO. If it's not feasible to make the program completely autonomous, then placement within a reporting structure to reduce conflict of interest and reduce intradepartmental competition for resources is best. This will reduce conflict of interest between competing goals in other departments that demand more return on investment criteria to show need for resources. It can also free up the food safety management program to identify food safety hazards within the business as its focus. For example, if the program is within or reports to the legal department, most decisions will likely be influenced due to fear of legal liability which could then reduce the effectiveness of the program to identify risk and then develop effective means to reduce them (e.g., records of risk not corrected/managed could reduce the desire to measure a risk especially if resources will not be made available to reduce them). It is true that documented knowledge of a risk, and not developing the means to address the risk, is a higher liability to the organization. However, I would argue the higher liability occurs when the risk is not measured and managed when there is clear evidence that risks are present (generally speaking, a significant number of hazards have been identified in all food processing and food retail sales businesses—see below). In fact, the new Food Safety Modernization Act of the United States (FSMA) will require businesses (all food manufactures) to identify hazards in their respective food production and demonstrate a plan to reduce these hazards in order to be compliant to this law. It is still important to seek inside (and sometimes outside) legal council before some hazard identification assessments are performed to protect the business from liability (e.g., when there is no industry standard for or regulatory requirement of prevention methods yet), but it is best to use this information (council) to make good decisions.

Another example: if the food safety management program is in/reports to the purchasing/supply chain department, then there could be conflict of interest between these two business functions. It is likely the supply chain/purchasing department has a mandate to seek the lowest price and best value and not to run out of product. The food safety management program's specifications of suppliers could increase some cost and limit supply if suppliers loose certification to provide products/ingredients to the organization or food safety issues drive product withdrawals of a suppliers product. Again, it is still important to closely partner with the supply chain/purchasing department and use information to make good decisions to ensure food safety at the lowest cost feasible. When the food safety management program is autonomous, it may provide unbiased recommendations to the organization using input from all stakeholders to enable better business decisions based on achieving the lowest known risk.

Once you have the food safety management program in the right place to enable it to objectively manage food safety, you need to structure the team's responsibilities around the three core business functions of the organization: supplier food safety, regulatory compliance, and retail food safety. The number of staff to manage the food safety of these three core business functions will most likely be based on several factors like the size of the organization (e.g., one million vs. one billion in sales), primary responsibilities owned by other departments (e.g., how many employees in other departments have shared responsibilities/roles vs. food safety subject matter expertise), complexity of the menu/products sold, volume of food produced in the supply chain (10 or 1,000 suppliers), and retail food production/sales (5 or 5,000 retail units) volume.

The key to an effective food safety management program organization will be found in each team member's influence on other departments and their primary focus on the three core functions of the business; supplier food safety (purchasing, food manufacturing, supplier quality, distribution), regulatory compliance (risk management, legal), and retail food safety (operations, human resources, public relations, equipment/facilities, and training). If the resources are available, the best structure would be one manager on the team with the responsibility and thus focus on each of these three core functions of the business (Fig. 3.1). Thus the manager responsible for the supplier food safety business functions would be responsible for setting systems/specifications, training/education requirements, production

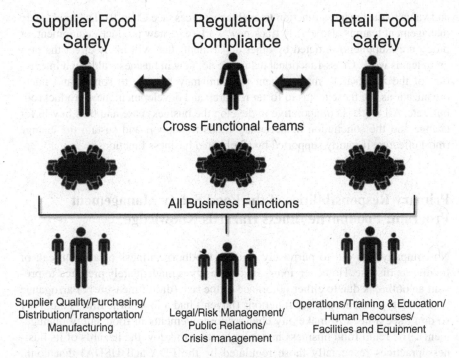

Fig. 3.1 Food safety management team organization with respective business function work

facilities requirements, and ensure execution and verification of each of these systems/specifications. Specific responsibilities would be designated for the manager over regulatory compliance and the manager over retail food safety respectively. Neglect of or less focus on any one business function area by a dedicated manager could increase risk to the business if the core function areas are complex (e.g., multiple perishable ingredients imported and distributed to multiple retail units in multiple states). If the food safety management program cannot support one manager for each business function area (e.g., if the business is small, has fewer products, has limited suppliers, or has only a few retail units), then whomever manages several core functions should have expertise in each to enable effective collaboration with other departments to achieve food safety program goals.

An effective method to expand the reach of the food safety management teams' impact is to enable participation (or develop and lead one if none exist) cross-functional teams centered around each of the three core business functions (usually multi-departmental). In this scenario, for example, the manager responsible for supplier food safety meets with the department team in the supply chain/purchasing and supplier quality departments at regular intervals. These meetings are purposely set to present risk and establish work needed to reduce these risks to the supply chain. The food safety management program can use these teams to introduce new work (new systems, projects, or food safety requirements) that impacts each core function area (and socialize the need within other departments) and enable joint study of the impact and value to the business function to enable resources (see Chap. 9). The food safety management team is also able to track new work (e.g., new products, equipment, or procedures/suppliers) initiated by other departments that will likely effect the program teams work. Cross-functional teams are not new in business (although integration of the food safety management program may be new to some), and many organizations use these teams to foster research and development, new product rollouts, etc. All work is collaborative to develop the business case and thus buy-in for change and the solicitation of necessary funds to support and sustain the change (most effective if jointly supported by all effected business functions).

Primary Responsibilities of the Food Safety Management Program: Foodborne Illness Hazards Knowledge

No company sets out to purposely cause a foodborne illness or an outbreak of foodborne disease. However, many find themselves inadequately prepared to prevent an outbreak due to either ignorance of the risk (didn't measure) or arrogance in the safety of their business functions (haven't had a foodborne illness outbreak so don't see a need to make any changes/improvements in food safety management). The retail food business has an obligation to know the hazards of its business practices (especially those regulated by the FDA and USDA) that could contribute to the risk of a foodborne illness (suppliers and retail food preparation) and implement controls for these hazards to ensure ignorance and arrogance are eliminated from the business. The first responsibility of the food safety management team therefore should be defining the food safety risks of the organizations operations using the knowledge of the hazards inherit in food production.

I attended a government-initiated conference (sponsored by the CDC/FDA, see Federal Register 2010) that was hosted to solicit input on the metrics needed to better attribute foodborne illness rates to their cause (e.g., failure to control the hazard) so the effectiveness of new intervention strategies (mostly regulatory controls on industry) could be better correlated to national disease rates. Tracking national disease rates by the CDC helps the FDA/USDA determine which regulatory intervention strategies (e.g., Juice HACCP) are working and which need additional development. When I was given the opportunity to speak to provide an industry perspective input, I performed an exercise with the audience (about 200 people) that started in this manner: I asked all the members of the audience to raise their hands IF they were ever an official member (part of a case control study) of a CDC investigated foodborne disease outbreak. I believe only one person raised their hand. However, when I asked the audience to raise their hands IF they were ever diagnosed with (or know for certain they had) a foodborne illness, the majority of the audience raised their hands. This exercise showed me (and them) that there are many foodborne illnesses that are not identified and counted by current disease surveillance systems, and thus, a food retail business cannot rely solely on reported disease rates and past information about what intervention strategies work best to prevent a foodborne illness. In fact, it is better to define risk (by investigating hazards within its own business functions) and developing cost effective prevention strategies before they are discovered.

Some food safety hazards present in food production were not previously identified until they became part of a multistate foodborne illness investigation. A good example of this can be found in the 2006 foodborne disease outbreak associated with fresh cut bagged spinach due to *E. coli* 0157 contamination (CDC 2006). This outbreak caused three deaths and over 200 illnesses that few businesses could have predicted based on the current knowledge of this hazard (and its probability) before the outbreak. Before this, although the fresh cut produce industry was aware of hazards associated with *E. coli* contamination, the majority of cases of foodborne disease outbreaks were associated with ground beef or other leafy greens like lettuce or tomatoes. The lesson here is that it is better to put resources to generate your own data on hazards from within all areas of the business (most importantly food production in suppliers facilities and retail units) to maximize prevention of a foodborne disease outbreak. If a hazard is identified but does not have a currently acceptable means (nor is it regulated) for prevention, then a system should be developed to reduce the probability of the hazard in the business function. Thus, knowledge of hazards should be a focus of the food safety management teams work on systems and specification design to avoid being part of a newly identified hazard in its business.

The CDC is the traditional source of foodborne disease knowledge as it investigates and then reports all multistate foodborne illness rates in the United States (note: outbreak investigations of infectious diseases effecting only one state are normally performed by the state and then reported to the CDC). Although significant foodborne illnesses are caused by chemical and physical contaminants in foods (the FDA and USDA report numerous recall actions every year on foods that are known to contain undeclared allergens or chemical/physical contamination), most of the well studied (but difficult to control) and thus reported causes of foodborne illnesses in the United States are those caused by microbial pathogens. Mead et al. (1999) published the first comprehensive estimates of the burden of foodborne diseases in the United States that to some seemed speculative (76 million illnesses a year, 325,000 hospitalizations, and 5,000 deaths) when only a small proportion of foodborne illnesses are confirmed by laboratory testing and reported to public health agencies each year. However, these often-cited data contributed to significant reform over the last 10 years in the regulatory systems (defined by the FDA and USDA) which were the result of additional academic and government studies, industry-based risk assessments, and additional CDC/FDA foodborne illness investigations that identified hazards within the food industry.

The CDC reported more recently on the national estimates of foodborne illnesses using more accurate statistical methods than were available in 1999. CDC now estimates that each year roughly 1 in 6 Americans (or 48 million people) acquire a foodborne illness, 128,000 are hospitalized, and 3,000 die of foodborne diseases (CDC 2011). The CDC reported that of all the top pathogens contributing to foodborne illnesses in the United States between 2000 to 2008, norovirus (often associated with

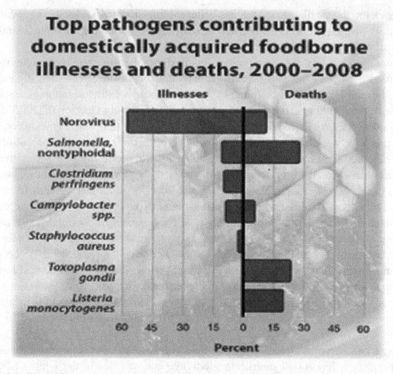

Fig. 3.2 Top pathogens contributing to domestically acquired foodborne illnesses and deaths, 2000–2008 (CDC 2012)

employee illnesses) cased the highest percentage of illnesses, while *Salmonella* (nontyphodial often associated with produce) caused the highest percentage of deaths (Fig. 3.2, CDC 2012). The CDC estimates that by reducing foodborne illness by only 10%, it would keep about five million Americans from getting sick each year.

Additional national foodborne disease rates were reported by Scallan et al. (2011) who provided a more precise estimate of the number and specific cause of microbial foodborne illnesses in the United States using laboratory-confirmed disease data primarily from the Foodborne Diseases Active Surveillance Network (FoodNet). Their data showed that each year, there are likely 9.4 million episodes of foodborne illness, 55,961 hospitalizations, and 1,351 deaths (many that could be prevented) caused by 31 known pathogens. More importantly, four pathogens (*Salmonella, E. coli* 0157:H7, *Listeria monocytogenes*, and *Campylobacter*) were reported to cause 21% of these diseases, 56% of hospitalizations, and 54% of foodborne disease deaths. These four pathogens are known to cause significant burden of disease as adulterates of beef, eggs, leafy greens, sprouts, and fish. Figure 3.3 shows additional attribution of foodborne illnesses in the United States, with poultry, leafy green produce, beef, and dairy foods contributing to the largest number of foodborne disease outbreaks over a 4-year period.

Fig. 3.3 Foods associated with foodborne disease outbreaks in the United States from 1,565 investigations over the of four years (CDC 2010)

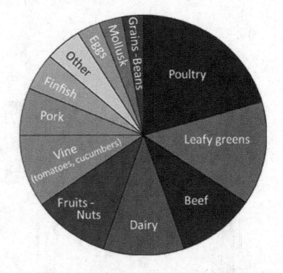

The economic burden of foodborne disease is high. In two recent follow-up studies to Scallan et al. (2011), an estimated annual cost of illness and quality-adjusted life years (QALY) loss in the United States due to these 31 pathogens was calculated. 14 pathogens were found to cause $14.0 billion in cost of illness and a loss of 61,000 QALYs (Hoffman et al. 2012), and poultry, produce, and complex manufactured foods were responsible for almost 60% of the total cost of illness and loss of QALYs (Batz et al. 2012) . Of these 14 pathogens, 5 pathogens were found to cause 90 % of total loss including nontyphodial *Salmonella enterica* ($3.3 billion), *Campylobacter* spp. ($1.7 billion), *Listeria monocytogenes* ($2.6 billion), *Toxoplasma gondii* ($3.0 Billion), and norovirus ($2 billion) (Hoffman et al. 2012). Cost of illness measurements are used in public policy analysis by the CDC, and these costs only estimate the burden of disease due to medical care and loss of an individual's public health (health state of an individual's comfort and ability to engage in normal activities). There are also significant associated cost to retail food businesses due to recall, claim investigations, loss sales, legal defense of claims, replacement of product, destruction of product, and indirect cost charged through increased cost of products and ingredients it purchases. A large percentage of this cost could be reduced by knowledge and prevention of these pathogens from contaminating food during manufacture or retail food preparation.

The most current data on foodborne illnesses associated to an individual food commodity can be found in the ongoing investigations and reports of the CDC and FDA. These investigations show us how these foodborne illnesses occur (e.g., how did the *E. coli* 0157:H7 bacteria get on the spinach) and the most likely methods to prevent them in the future. The CDC developed a new public web site called FoodCORE (see Fig. 3.4) in 2011 (the CORE stands for Centers for Outbreak Response Enhancement; see: http://www.cdc.gov/foodcore/) that now reports the most current information on ongoing foodborne illness investigations as they occur each year. This web site can be used to monitor similar commodity-related issues

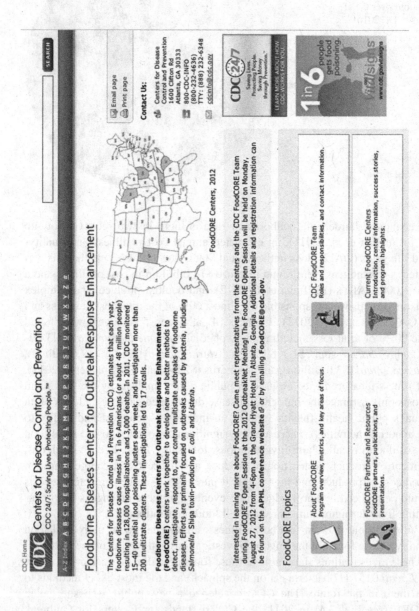

Fig. 3.4 Source for the most current foodborne disease outbreak investigations in the United States at CDC's FoodCORE website (http://www.cdc.gov/foodcore/index.html)

(sometimes even before the FDA/USDA initiates recalls on a product) to learn what hazards most likely lead to the outbreak of disease.

The retail food business and its manufacturers have a public health responsibility to protect their customers from foodborne disease illnesses. In fact, I would argue that this industry has a greater responsibility than regulatory agencies due to its knowledge of the specific processes and procedures of its food production and potential food safety hazards in these (e.g., measured by audits, finished product testing, undeclared allergen use, environmental sampling, cleaning, and sanitation validations) that could contribute to a foodborne illness. The focus of the remaining chapters of this book will be on the design of the systems, training/education, facilities, execution/verification, and influence/resources necessary to control hazards in the supplier (purchasing, food manufacturing, distribution) regulatory (risk management, legal), and retail (operations, human resources, public relations, equipment/facilities, and training) functions of a food retail business. The public health responsibility shared with public health professionals can be enhanced via partnerships with public health officials as discussed in Chap. 10.

References

Batz et al (2012) Ranking the disease burden of 14 pathogens in food sources in the United States using Attribution data from outbreak investigations and expert elicitation. J Food Prot 75:1288–1291

CDC (2006) Multi-State Outbreak of E. coli O157:H7 Infections From Spinach, September–October 2006. Available via internet at http://www.cdc.gov/ecoli/2006/september/

CDC (2010) CDC Estimates of Foodborne Illness in the United States. Available via internet at http://www.cdc.gov/foodborneburden/cdc-and-food-safety.html

CDC (2011) 2011 Estimates of Foodborne Illness in the United States. Available via internet at http://www.cdc.gov/Features/dsFoodborneEstimates/

CDC (2012) 2011 Estimates of Foodborne Illness in the United States. Available via internet at http://www.cdc.gov/Features/dsFoodborneEstimates/

Federal Register (2010) Measuring progress on food safety: current status and future directions; public workshop. Department of Health and Human Services, Food and Drug Administration. Available via internet at http://www.fda.gov/food/newsevents/workshopsmeetingsconferences/ucm201102.htm

Hoffman et al (2012) Annual cost of illness and quality-adjusted life year losses in the United States due to 14 foodborne pathogens. J Food Prot 75:1292–1302

Mead PS et al (1999) Food related illness and death in the United States. Emerg Infect Dis 5:607–524

Scallan E et al (2011) Foodborne illness acquired in the United States- major pathogens. Emerg Infect Dis Vol 17(1):7–15

Yiannas F (2009) Food safety culture; creating a behavior-based food safety management system. Springer, Heidelberg

Chapter 4
Systems

The foundation for a successful food safety management program will be found in the risk-based systems defined to reduce hazards that are known to cause a foodborne illness. Systems can be defined as programs/policies and standard operation procedures (SOPs) that support the management of food safety hazards within the organization. Before these systems can be implemented, the food safety management team must define the hazards in all of its business functions. Thankfully, there is a large volume of information from government, academia, and national and international organizations on what the *hazards* are in the manufacture and retail sale of food. Once the hazards have been defined within each of the business functions (e.g., restaurant food prep of each menu item or supplier production of an ingredient or product), the team should develop and implement systems that are proven to reduce the risk of these hazards. Again, a large volume of information on effective *preventative measures* is available and continues to be updated by government, academia, and national and international organizations.

The key to sustaining systems within a food retail business (because all systems cost money) will be found in the balance between the cost of the system and its value in preventing a hazard vs. the cost of not implementing the system. Traditionally, the costs of prevention many food retail organizations look at are the predicted cost of a foodborne illness litigation (which can be in the millions of dollars) and brand name reputation (lost sales due to lost customer confidence) if there is a foodborne illness claim or investigation by regulatory authorities. However, true cost (and reduced profit) is inherent in the organization due to manufacturing defects (all food manufacturing has defects that can lead to product withdrawals or recall), and money spent on reducing defects in food manufacturing and food prep at the retail level will likely prevent many food safety hazards as well. The right systems provide the platform for continuous verification of hazard prevention and can provide knowledge to the organization to make good decisions during management of product defect investigations and food safety claims made by customers and/or regulatory authorities.

H. King, *Food Safety Management: Implementing a Food Safety Program in a Food Retail Business*, Food Microbiology and Food Safety, DOI 10.1007/978-1-4614-6205-7_4,
© Springer Science+Business Media New York 2013

Importance of Systems

The role of systems is to ensure management of hazards in a food retail business. Well-defined food safety systems can help the team make both good business decisions (protecting the bottom line) and public health decisions (protect its customers). Let me illustrate this concept with this scenario and the decisions made based on the presence or absence of defined food safety systems. Suppose you receive a call from your 1–800 customer service agency on Saturday afternoon that a customer called and said the chocolate milk her child drank tasted like it had chemicals in it, and the customer was calling while on the way to the hospital with the child. Chocolate milk sales in your retail chain average half a million bottles a day. If you pulled (recall) all the chocolate milk (e.g., if you can't identify which lot/batch is effected) from your retail stores, your chain likely will lose $250,000 a day in profit (if the claim is false, a significant loss to the business). However, if you don't recall the affected milk you decide to wait and see before you initiate a recall more children may be poisoned if the milk is contaminated with a chemical. *If* you have the proper systems in place (each system/specification is identified below), this might be the likely decisions you can make of this scenario:

Day One:

(a) Follow up with the customer immediately to see how the child is doing and request if chocolate milk packaging is available (obtain lot/batch information via photo identification if possible). Call the retail unit where the product was sold to identify the lot/batch sold today and have this unit stop sales, hold this product (mark as "not for service, see manager"), and seek replacement/credit. Customer says child is OK and does not appear sick, but she took child to obtain poison control council just in case. Request to obtain the product from the customer if customer will allow for testing (this could help quickly identify any possible chemical contaminants; chain of custody will be established). Product is obtained from customer by the retail unit personnel who sold the product, lot/batch identified, and customers product, and a case of product from the same retail store is sent to third-party contract laboratory for testing (biological and chemical). See *f* below for final results in this scenario. Continue to monitor customer surveillance system carefully for any further claims for the next hour. *Systems/specifications*: *customer surveillance system, supplier finished product specification* (*lot/batch-date/time identification*), *product traceability system, crisis response system*, and *ingredient/product defect investigation system* (chain of custody procedures for product retrieval/investigations and customer claims, contract laboratory approved for ingredient/product testing).

(b) Initiate a product withdrawal at the retail level (communicated to all units unless you know which units only received the effected lot/batch). All retail units quarantine lot/batch of product on-site and do not sell until notice from the food safety management team. *Systems/specifications*: *ingredient/product withdrawal/recall system* (to contact all or designated units and document compliance to withdrawal notice (within 2 h)), *supplier finished product specification* (*lot/batch-date/time identification*), *and product traceability system.*

(c) Call your distributors and initiate a product hold of the exact lot/batch of chocolate milk to ensure no more product is transported to the retail units. Product is to be quarantined until further notice. *Systems/specifications: product traceability system* and *distributor finished product handling/transportation specification* (for quarantining/storage of ingredient/product on-site to prevent delivery to units).

(d) Because your chocolate milk supplier was required to retain representative samples of each lot/batch of finished product, you request supplier data immediately, but also send these samples to be retested to show there were no clean in place (CIP) errors (i.e., chemical or biological contamination) by third-party laboratory as confirmation. Have records of what chemicals are used in all CIP systems for this manufacturer. Request supplier to investigate all production records to validate food safety systems were in compliance and approved chemicals only used for CIP. You discover that tested product lot/batch at supplier and third-party laboratory showed no chemicals detected. *Systems/specifications: prerequisite specifications for supplier, product traceability system, supplier finished product specification, ingredient/product defect investigation system.*

(e) No other customers have reported issues in last few hours (via customer surveillance system) and more specifically from original retail unit, and customer reports child is not sick. All retained sample data for chemical analysis is negative. Product remains on hold at retail and distribution levels (i.e., no product is allowed to be sold) until final laboratory test confirm negative data. *Systems/ specifications: customer surveillance system ingredient/product defect investigation system.*

Day Two:

(f) The customers product tested positive for *Lactobacillus* spp. (a spoilage organism that can cause milk to have a chemical off-flavor) but no chemical contaminants, and customer's child is ok (never became ill). Distributors and retail units are contacted to take product off hold/withdrawal and resume deliveries and sales. *Systems/specifications: ingredient/product withdrawal/recall system* (to contact all or designated retail units that product can be sold) and *distributor finished product handling/transportation specification* for release of quarantined ingredient/product back into distribution.

Because of the systems you have in place, you are able to make these business decisions while also being prepared to make the proper public health decisions if necessary (e.g., if child is reported to be sick, additional customers reported illness, and/or retained sample data shows biological or chemical contamination). The only safe decision to make without any systems/specifications in place in this scenario (and more likely still if the customer reported the child was ill or additional customers reported illness) is to recall all chocolate milk from all retail units immediately (assuming you have a recall system) and follow up with distributors and manufacturer to try and prevent delivery of the product to retail units.

Systems Development: Identifying Hazards and Determining Risk

Before the most appropriate risk-based systems can be designed and implemented, the food safety management team must determine the food safety hazards in all of its business functions and then estimate the probability of these hazards to define their risk. Food safety risk can most simply be defined by the equation:

$$\text{Hazard} \times \text{Probability} = \text{Risk}$$

Both a hazard and a probability must be present in order for there to be a risk. It is best to determine if a hazard is present and probable first before attempting to develop control systems to reduce a presumed risk within a business function. It is not recommended to ignore hazards in this equation when determining whether there is risk, because even if probability is very low, a moderate hazard may be deemed too high a risk. This simple risk equation can serve as a means to determine priority of risk and thus systems that need to be developed to reduce the highest risk first (discussed in more detail in Chap. 9 as they relate to seeking resources). Of course this risk definition is not the best means to calculate the severity of a hazard, but it can quickly define the need for systems/specifications since both hazards and probability must exist in order for there to be a risk.

It may be necessary to perform a more formal risk analysis to determine how best to manage, assess, and communicate the risk in order to ensure the hazard has been controlled (also discussed in more detail in Chap. 9). Risk analysis is not a uniform process, and it has much iteration based on who describes it, who uses it, and how it can be calculated. Some probabilities of hazards (risk) may be very low under current circumstances but change quickly when circumstances change (e.g., adding a new complex menu item to retail units or when a manufacturer adds more ingredients to a production line). Generally speaking, most hazards in food manufacture and retail food prep (due to the dangers inherit in the contamination of foods) should be controlled and reevaluated regularly to see if probability has changed if not controlled.

Let's go back to the example in Chap. 2 with the difficult to maintain sanitizer solution, and Sara the restaurant owners method to prevent this risk in her restaurant; now in the context of risk definition. If you will recall, using cloth reusable towels (stored in the proper strength of sanitizer) to clean food contact surfaces reduces cross contamination of food (the hazard depends on what pathogens and how many are likely found in the restaurant, e.g., if raw hamburger meat is prepared). When the probability of improper sanitizer solution is high (employees do not maintain the proper solution strength), the risk of cross contamination is high (high hazard × high probability = high risk). Say, for example, Sara innovated a means to reduce the probability of this high hazard by an improved means to train and educate her employees to maintain the sanitizer solution (one that was verified to work) rather than developing a new disposable sanitizing cloth (that could be more cost to her restaurant). Because the hazard can be controlled by a strong food safety advocate who ensures training and education is verified, this may be a better economic decision for the business to control risk.

However, say that Sara's restaurant is part of a chain of hamburger restaurants, and the corporate headquarters' studies, and finds 85% of the restaurants do not maintain the proper sanitizer strength even with enhanced training/education tools provided (even higher risk to the retail business). In this case, a better decision would be to implement a system (e.g., new standard operating procedures—SOPs) to reduce the risk (requiring disposable sanitizing wipes rather than allowing use of reusable cloth towels) throughout the chain.

The food safety management team should measure risk in the two major components of the business, the supply chain (where ingredients and products are produced and delivered to the retail units through a distribution system) and food production and sales in its retail units (where ingredients and products are prepared, packaged, and sold to customers). A large number of food commodities in manufacturing and retail production have been extensively studied by government, academia, and industry to determine hazards and their probability in the cause of foodborne illnesses and the means to reduce these hazards by specific intervention methods (e.g., a hazard in milk production are microbial pathogens that can be present in raw milk which are eliminated by heat pasteurization). However, most food production (including within a retail food establishment) has many variables that can create new hazards due to the normal business needs and change within the organization (e.g., change in packaging of a product for retail sales, increased sales and thus production in older facilities, change in procedures due to change in equipment, suppliers making changes to their food production lines to accommodate additional buyers of new products, etc.). The food safety management team must therefore continually measure food production in its own facilities and suppliers for new hazards in all business functions of their organization.

Systems Development: Manufacture and Corporate Control Systems

There are two types of systems to control hazards (Table 4.1) that a food retail business should develop to ensure food safety. The first one I will call a *manufacture control system*. *Manufacture control systems* are systems/specifications that control hazards that occur at the lowest level of food manufacturing and retail food prep (e.g., cooking temperature requirement to kill microbial pathogens in raw foods, finished product specification). The second type of systems to control hazards I will call *corporate control systems*. These systems/specifications are cross functional within the food retail business that control more complex hazards within and across business functions (usually those with a higher degree of probability/exposure like a defective product that is distributed to all the retail units under the food retail business's management). It is not the scope of this chapter to cover all the systems used to control hazards in supplier and retail components of the organization, but I will discuss those that are known to be most effective and briefly provide examples of how the food safety management program should use them.

Table 4.1 Example manufacture and corporate control systems necessary for hazard control managed by the food safety management program

Manufacture control systems	Corporate control systems
Prerequisite specifications—suppliers	Crisis preparedness and response
Prerequisite specifications—retail units	Supplier certification and verification
Supplier HACCP	Retail unit specification verification
Retail unit HACCP	Product traceability
Supplier finished product specifications—recipes/ procedures (also see Fig. 4.6)	Customer surveillance and response
Retail unit finished product specifications—recipes/ procedures	Product defect surveillance—supply chain
Distribution finished product handling/transportation specification	Ingredient/product defect investigations and resolution
Product defect reporting—retail	Product withdrawal/recall communications and compliance
Distribution/transportation temperature control	Document control and records
Education specifications of retail employees/supplier employees	Education specifications of corporate staff

Manufacture Control Systems

HACCP

The most well-known *manufacture control system* in the food business is HACCP (hazard analysis and critical control point). HACCP is the most effective system to control hazards at the manufacture level because it relies on continuous monitoring and control of critical control points (CCPs) along the production and processing continuum in all manufacturing of food (in supplier, distributor, and retail components of the business). CCPs are the points where loss of control would result in an unsafe product or more specifically as the points in food manufacture "where the identified hazard(s) may be prevented from entering the food, eliminated from it, or reduced to acceptable levels" (Stevenson and Bernard 1995).

HACCP is a preventative food safety assurance system that provides the most value to a food retail business because it catches the hazard and makes corrective action mandatory before a product is finished (less cost to the business) as opposed to a nontraditional corrective system that measures the presence of a hazard in the finished product. Because HACCP is such an effective means to control hazards in food manufacturing, both the USDA and FDA have established HACCP as a mandated national food regulation for all food manufacturing in the United States (FSIS 1996 and 21 C.F.R. part 114 in Federal Registry, respectively). HACCP is also a recognized system in international food trade even though it is voluntary (CAC 1997). Food safety managers should have a strong competency in the practice of these principles, but if not, the best place to start to learn and develop methods to

APPENDIX C

Examples of Questions to be Considered When Conducting a Hazard Analysis

The hazard analysis consists of asking a series of questions which are appropriate to the process under consideration. The purpose of the questions is to assist in identifying potential hazards.

A. I ngredients
  1. Does the food contain any sensitive ingredients thatmay present microbiological hazards (e.g., Salmonella, Staphylococcus aureus); chemical hazards (e.g., aflatoxin, antibiotic or pesticide residues); or physical hazards (stones, glass, metal)?
  2. Are potable water, ice and steam used in formulating orin handling the food?
  3. What are the sources (e.g., geographical region, specific supplier)
B. Intrinsic Factors-Physical characteristics and composition (e.g., pH, type of acidulants, fermentable carbohydrate, water activity, preservatives) of the food during and after processing.
  1. What hazards may resultifthe food composition is notcontrolled?
  2. Does the food permit survival or multiplication of pathogens and/or toxin formation in the food during processing?
  3. Will the food permit survival or multiplication of pathogens and/or toxin formation during subsequent steps in the food chain?
  4. Are there other similar products in the market place? What has been the safety record for these products? What hazards have been associated with the products?
C. Procedures used for processing
  1. Does the process include a controllable processing step that destroys pathogens? If so,which pathogens? Consider both vegetative cells and spores.
  2. Ifthe product is subject to recontamination between processing (e.g., cooking, pasteurizing) and packaging which biological, chemical or physical hazards are likely to occur?
D. Microbial content of the food
  1. What is the normal microbial content of the food?
  2. Does the microbial population change during the normaltime the food is stored priorto consumption?
  3. Does the subsequent change in microbial population alter the safety of the food?
  4. Do the answers to the above questions indicate a high likelihood ofcertain biologicalhazards?
E. Facility design
  1. Does the layout of the facility provide an adequate separation of raw materials from ready-to-eat (RTE) foods if this is important to food safety? If not,what hazards should be considered as possible contaminants of the RTE products?
  2. Is positive air pressure maintained in product packaging areas? Is this essential for product safety?
  3. Is the traffic pattern forpeople and moving equipment a significant source of contamination?
F. Equipment design and use
  1. Will the equipment provide the time-temperature control that is necessary for safe food?
  2. Is the equipment properly sized for the volume offood that will be processed?
  3. Can the equipment be sufficiently controlled so that the variation in performance will be within the tolerances required to produce a safe food?
  4. Is the equipment reliable oris it prone to frequentbreakdowns?
  5. Is the equipment designed so that it can be easily cleaned and sanitized?
  6. Is there a chance for product contamination with hazardous substances; e.g., glass?
  7. What product safety devices are used to enhance consumersafety?
     - metal detectors
     - magnets
     - sifters
     - filters
     - screens
     - thermometers
     - bone removal devices
     - dud detectors
  8. To what degree will normal equipment wear affect the likely occurrence of a physical hazard (e g , metal) in the product?
  9. Are allergen protocols needed in using equipment for different products?

Fig. 4.1 Development of a HACCP system. Hazard analysis and critical control points principles and application guidelines (partial list); National advisory committee on microbiological criteria for foods (FDA 1997)

apply them is with the FDA retail food protection site on HACCP applications in retail foods (FDA 1997). Figure 4.1 shows a series of questions the FDA recommends as a means to assist in the identification of hazards in a food manufacturing facility (supply level) and a CCP decision tree to assist manufactures with control measure development for each hazard. All suppliers to a retail food business should be required to provide a HACCP plan for any product manufactured for the business,

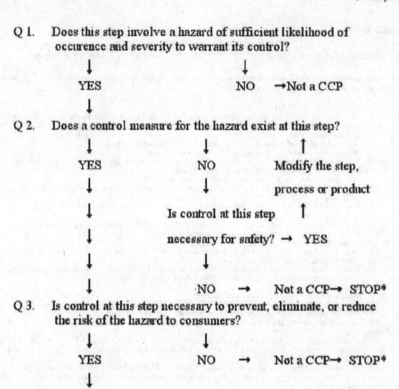

Q 1.   Does this step involve a hazard of sufficient likelihood of
       occurence and severity to warrant its control?

          ↓   ↓
          YES   NO   →Not a CCP
          ↓

Q 2.   Does a control measure for the hazard exist at this step?

          ↓   ↓   ↑
          YES   NO   Modify the step,
          ↓   ↓   process or product
          ↓   Is control at this step   ↑
          ↓   necessary for safety? →   YES
          ↓   ↓
          ↓   ·NO   →   Not a CCP→ STOP*

Q 3.   Is control at this step necessary to prevent, eliminate, or reduce
       the risk of the hazard to consumers?

          ↓   ↓
          YES   NO   →   Not a CCP→ STOP*
          ↓
          CCP

* Proceed to next step in the process.

Fig. 4.1 (continued)

and the food safety management team should be able to review and verify the CCPs within this plan during manufacture of its products (to be discussed in more detail in Chap. 7). The new Food Safety Modernization Act will soon require that all food manufacturers identify their hazards and the methods they use to prevent them (FDA 2012b). For a more detailed application of HACCP as a *manufacture control system* at the supplier level (helpful to identify microbial pathogen hazards and control during food manufacturing), I recommend the *Scientific criteria to ensure safe food* by the Institute of Medicine, National Research Council (2003) and *Microbiological risk assessment in food processing* (Brown and Stringer 2002).

HACCP is also used, although less often and more on a voluntary basis, in food service and retail establishments. The FDA has identified many of the most common hazards (Fig. 4.2) and has listed many of the recommended CCPs, CPs (control points), and control measures based on extensive studies shown to reduce risk within the retail and food service industry and its manual on managing food safety using HACCP is an important tool for applying this system in retail operations (FDA 2006, 2009a). The most common CCPs in retail food preparation are found in cooking, cooling, and cold and hot holding of food outside of the temperature

Annex 4, Table 1. Selected Biological Hazards Found at Retail, Associated Foods, and Control Measures		
HAZARD	**ASSOCIATED FOODS**	**CONTROL MEASURES**
Bacteria		
Bacillus cereus (intoxication caused by heat stable, preformed emetic toxin and infection by heat labile, diarrheal toxin)	Meat, poultry, starchy foods (rice, potatoes), puddings, soups, cooked vegetables	Cooking, cooling, cold holding, hot holding
Campylobacter jejuni	Poultry, raw milk	Cooking, handwashing, prevention of cross-contamination
Clostridium botulinum	Vacuum-packed foods, reduced oxygen packaged foods, under-processed canned foods, garlic-in-oil mixtures, time/temperature abused baked potatoes/sautéed onions	Thermal processing (time + pressure), cooling, cold holding, hot holding, acidification and drying, etc.
Clostridium perfringens	Cooked meat and poultry, Cooked meat and poultry products including casseroles, gravies	Cooling, cold holding, reheating, hot holding
E. coli O157:H7 (other shiga toxin-producing E. coli)	Raw ground beef, raw seed sprouts, raw milk, unpasteurized juice, foods contaminated by infected food workers via fecal-oral route	Cooking, no bare hand contact with RTE foods, employee health policy, handwashing, prevention of cross-contamination, pasteurization or treatment of juice
Listeria monocytogenes	Raw meat and poultry, fresh soft cheese, paté, smoked seafood, deli meats, deli salads	Cooking, date marking, cold holding, handwashing, prevention of cross-contamination
Salmonella spp.	Meat and poultry, seafood, eggs, raw seed sprouts, raw vegetables, raw milk, unpasteurized juice	Cooking, use of pasteurized eggs, employee health policy, no bare hand contact with RTE foods, handwashing, pasteurization or treatment of juice
Shigella spp.	Raw vegetables and herbs, other foods contaminated by infected workers via fecal-oral route	Cooking, no bare hand contact with RTE foods, employee health policy, handwashing
Staphylococcus aureus (preformed heat stable toxin)	RTE PHF foods touched by bare hands after cooking and further time/temperature abused	Cooling, cold holding, hot holding, no bare hand contact with RTE food, handwashing
Vibrio spp.	Seafood, shellfish	Cooking, approved source, prevention of cross-contamination, cold holding
Parasites		
Anisakis simplex	Various fish (cod, haddock, fluke, pacific salmon, herring, flounder, monkfish)	Cooking, freezing
Taenia spp.	Beef and pork	Cooking
Trichinella spiralis	Pork, bear, and seal meat	Cooking
Viruses		
Hepatitis A and E	Shellfish, any food contaminated by infected worker via fecal-oral route	Approved source, no bare hand contact with RTE food, minimizing bare hand contact with foods not RTE, employee health policy, handwashing
Other Viruses (Rotavirus, Norovirus, Reovirus)	Any food contaminated by infected worker via fecal-oral route	No bare hand contact with RTE food, minimizing bare hand contact with foods not RTE, employee health policy, handwashing
RTE = ready-to-eat		
PHF = potentially hazardous food (time/temperature control for safety food)		

Fig. 4.2 Common hazards and control measures in retail food establishments (FDA 2009a)

danger zone (41 °F–135 °F; where pathogens grow best in food). Some states require HACCP in the retail food service establishment and provide a template for retail establishments to indicate a HACCP plan for each food item prepared. For example, the state of Maryland requires HACCP plans to be created and certified annually (Maryland Department of Health and Mental Hygiene 2008), and CCPs and training documentation are checked during regular health inspections (Fig. 4.3). These templates provide a good starting point to measure hazards and set CCPs to control these hazards in the retail food environment. There are also other organizations that provide a service to develop a HACCP program for a food retail business (and for suppliers as well). These organizations can be found very easily on the internet, and the personnel in these organizations have a great deal of prior experience in HACCP development (usually former academic or government scientist).

Some food manufacturing control at the retail level may seem to be more difficult when you try to establish well-defined CCPs when there is no direct means to eliminate a pathogen or reduce them to acceptable (assume safe) levels. However, the HACCP

HACCP Plan Form (Example 1)

Facility: ABC Restaurant   Preparer: CDE Consultants   Date: 00/00/00

Food item: Beef Roast / Sliced Beef

Flow diagram or descriptive narrative of the food preparation steps for the food item:

Receive Frozen ⇨ Thaw ⇨ Cook ⇨ Hot Hold ⇨ Slice ⇨ Serve ⇨ Discard
                         CCP 1   CCP 2

Discard ⇦ Serve ⇦ Slice ⇦ Reheat ⇦ Cool
                    CCP 4   CCP 3

HACCP Chart

Critical Control Points (CCPs)	Monitoring Procedures	Corrective Actions
1. **Cook** to internal temperature of 145°F for a minimum of 3 minutes	Check the temperature of the product's center with a calibrated stem thermometer	Continue to cook
2. **Hot Hold** at minimum of 140°F (Maximum of 4 hours)	Check the internal temperature of the product every hour	If internal temp. is less than 140°F for more than 1 hr. - Discard. If internal temp. is less than 140°F for 1 hr. or less, rapidly reheat to 165°F for 15 seconds.
3. **Cool** so that internal temperature is less than 70°F in 2 hrs., and less than 45°F in an additional 4 hrs.	Check the internal temperature of the product at one hour intervals	Discard product
4. **Reheat** to internal temperature of 165°F for at least 15 seconds	Check the internal temperature of the product	Discard product if it fails to reach 165°F within 2 hours

Equipment Utilized at each Critical Control Point (include type and quantity of each unit)

CCP 1: Convection Oven (2)

CCP 2: Heat Lamps (4)

CCP 3: Walk-in Cooler (1)

CCP 4: Convection Oven (2)

Fig. 4.3 Example HACCP development plan for food production in a retail food service establishment (Maryland and HACCP 2008)

development process can still produce a reduction in a hazard and its probability if not eliminated completely. Fresh served raw produce (where there is no kill step) is a good example of this challenge. Removing and discarding the outer leaves of leafy green produce (e.g., whole head iceberg lettuce) before rinsing could remove and possibly reduce to acceptable levels those pathogens that may have contaminated the produce before it is received by a restaurant. In fact, studies performed on these types of bulk leafy green produce showed a 1-log reduction (or 90%) of total bacteria from the produce using this method (unpublished data).

Likewise, other studies have shown that when different types of produce (lettuce, broccoli, cantaloupe, spinach, and green onions) is rinsed with running tap water, another 0.5–1.5-log reduction of *Escherichia coli* 0157.H7, *Listeria monocytogenes*, and *Salmonella enterica* is achieved (Parish et al. 2003; Fishburn et al. 2012) and interestingly a 2-log reduction on tomatoes (Fishburn et al. 2012). Although making these two actions (removal of outer leaves (CCP-1) and rinsing in running tap water (CCP-2)), each CCP may not perfectly fit the HACCP definition (primarily because most raw produce is not contaminated with pathogens nor are there any predictive models for how many pathogens are expected to be found on different produce types), verifying these CCPs could be speculated to eliminate the hazard if a low dose (likely less than 2–3 log, my speculation based on review of the scientific literature) contaminate was on the leafy green produce at any time.

This concept of using HACCP principals to reduce risk (unknown probabilities of known hazards; e.g., degree of bacterial contamination expected to be found on bulk leafy green produce) made me interested (as others have been for many years as evidenced by the scientific literature published on this subject, reviewed by the FDA 2009b) in working toward the development of an improved CCP for produce rinse at the retail level. Working with the University of Georgia Center for Food Safety (funded by the USDA and my retail business), we tested the efficacy of using electrolyzed water (Panglol et al. 2009) to kill *E. coli* 0157 pathogens inoculated on the most common raw produce (mostly used to make salads) prepared from bulk in a typical restaurant. Electrolyzed water was chosen due to its chemical safety (it associates back into H_2O after treatment), and our internal research showing it had the least amount of effect on product taste/color. Although the variability of log reduction of *E. coli* was high between produce types (a 7-log reduction was achieved on lemons but only 1-log reduction on cabbage), there was consistent removal and killing of the *E. coli* in the rinse water (perhaps enabling a soak of the produce to enhance killing of *E. coli* via exposure time). Increasing time of exposure and soak with fresh electrolyzed water would be expected to further reduce *E. coli*. Of course, other pathogens most commonly found on produce would need to be studied. Other groups have more extensively studied different chemical treatment of produce as a means to eliminate the hazard of pathogen contamination (literature reviewed by the FDA 2009b). More recently, Fishburn et al. (2012), also from the University of Georgia showed that electrolyzed water treatment of lettuce, broccoli, cantaloupe, spinach, and green onions showed more consistent effectiveness reducing *E. coli* 0157.H7, *L. monocytogenes*, and *S. enterica* on these produce than ozone, a commercial vegetable wash, or tap water. A chemical treatment of produce as a new CCP should be developed for retail food service establishments to enhance a HACCP plan for produce preparation. This would enable a more uniform kill step for produce while protecting its nutritional value; enhancing its use in products on the menu in restaurants and other retail establishments.

Not all *manufacture control systems* are based on HACCP (i.e., not defined with a CP or CCP) but may be just as effective as HACCP in indirectly or directly preventing hazards. Some additional important manufacture control systems are listed in Table 4.1. Two important systems necessary to reduce risk and ensure product integrity (and less defects) in both supplier and retail environments are prerequisite specifications and finished product specifications.

Prerequisite Specifications

A prerequisite specification is defined as the steps or procedures that control the operational conditions within a food establishment and promote environmental conditions that are favorable for the production of safe food. For example, an equipment maintenance program describes the activities that must be performed to prevent deterioration of equipment which can lead to physical, biological, or chemical hazards. The FDA has well-established prerequisite specifications called GMPs (good manufacturing practices) published in Title 21 of the Code of Federal Regulations, Part 110 (CFR 2011). According to the FDA, "GMPs describe the methods, equipment, facilities, and controls for producing processed food". As the minimum sanitary and processing requirements for producing safe and wholesome food, they are an important part of regulatory control over the safety of the nation's food supply. GMPs also serve as the basis for FDA regulatory compliance inspections of food manufactures. The most current GMPs are the result of many years of research and investigations into the hazards leading to foodborne disease outbreaks in the United States and their controls. Because the FDA inspects most food manufacturing facilities against GMPs, the majority of third-party auditing firms have established GMP-based food safety audits, and these audits have been used by most food retail businesses as a means to verify prerequisite specifications of its suppliers.

A more recent application of industry initiated prerequisite specifications (like FDAs, GMPs, and audits of GMPs) can be found in the Global Food Safety Initiative (GFSI). The Global Food Safety Initiative is a business-driven trade group set up for the continuous improvement of food safety management control systems. GFSI provides a platform for collaboration of the world's leading food safety experts from retailer, manufacturer, and food service companies globally, on setting feasible food safety standards. The GFSI was launched in 2000 with members collaborating in numerous technical working groups to study and set standards for current food safety issues defined by GFSI stakeholders. Current work in GFSI include setting the industry standards for food safety requirements along the entire food supply chain that covers feed, distribution, and packaging.

GFSI guidance documents (which are similar to FDA guidance documents) are based on the current edition of the CODEX alimentarius commission guidelines for the application of the hazard analysis and critical control point (HACCP) system and the National Advisory Committee on Microbiological Criteria for Foods (NACMCF) Hazard Analysis and Critical Control Point Principles and Application Guidelines, adopted August 14, 1997. These guidance documents serve as a platform for development of prerequisite specifications (GMPs) that are specific to all areas of food production including manufacturing and farms. There are currently nine schemes approved to enable certification via supplier facility audits (each facility must achieve certification independently of the parent business) and include the BRC Global Standard for Food Safety, CanadaGAP, FSSC 22000 Food Products, Global Aquaculture Alliance Seafood Processing Standard, Global G.A.P, Global Red Meat Standard, IFS, PrimusGFS, and Safe Quality Food (SQF).

Retail food businesses can select certified (GFSI compliant) suppliers (or require certification as a prerequisite program) with the confidence that these faculties meet defined food safety prerequisite specifications which are certified annually through approved auditing firms. The benefits to the buyer are that they can trust this certification as evidence of a well-defined food safety prerequisite specification in the certified food manufacturing facility or farm. The buyer can add addendums specific to its ingredients/ product production to this prerequisite specification, for example, allergen testing requirement after cleaning and sanitation, which are then audited by the auditing firms during the certification audits. The benefits to the suppliers are in the acceptance of this certification audit by multiple buyers reducing the cost of individual and often times different prerequisite specification audits in their facilities. Many firms also help suppliers work toward improvements to gain GFSI certification (which helps them grow their business); many retail food businesses only accept GFSI certified suppliers. Figure 4.4 shows an example of the minimum requirements that must be defined for a manufacturing facility contracted to make products for a food retail business, under SQF certification, a GFSI accredited scheme. Many of these elements are in FDA GMP specifications based on the type of food produced by the facility and the level of certification. A prerequisite program should be expected for all suppliers to a food retail business.

Prerequisite specifications can also be defined for each retail facility (usually called a retail plan requirement by the state regulatory authority and are often required in order to obtain a food service permit). The guides provided by these states are the best source for establishing a retail facility prerequisite specification (before design and construction) to ensure retail permit acceptance in each state. Most are based on the FDA retail plan requirement and can be easily found on the web site of the state regulatory agency tasked to permit food retail and food service establishments (in much greater detail there), and include elements shown in Fig. 4.5. Once general guidelines are established and the current menu is known, it is best to develop more specific guidelines for the safe flow of food in each facility to ensure retail environments are conducive to the production of safe food with the least amount of risk for cross contamination (facilities design is discussed in more detail in Chap. 6). Knowledge of the prerequisite specifications for the menu in retail stores should be the foundation of the retail business facilities design and construction departments work.

Finished Product Specifications

All manufactured ingredient and products have defects no matter how well a organization attempts to prevent product defects. The food safety management program should focus its resources therefore on ensuring any defect is not a food safety hazard but would only affect the quality of the ingredient/product (of course the quality program would work to reduce these defects as well). Thus, another manufacture control system important to ensure food safety of the ingredients and products produced for a food retail business and the products produced in its retail units is a finished product specification for each product. Many products manufactured specifically for a retail food business may be perishable (no preservatives, and thus require refrigeration as the primary means to sustain quality and food safety of the product) or have minimum secondary processing at the retail unit (e.g., maintaining cold by refrigeration or cooking to prepare or hold product for service). Therefore, it is important to establish and document clearly defined ingredient list and concentrations, clearly defined procedures on how to make the product, and clearly defined food safety requirements written into the procedures (e.g., CCPs that must be checked) in the life cycle of the product (during manufacture, distribution, and food preparation for service and sale at retail).

Finished product specifications for ingredient/product manufacturers are more easily established because the manufacturer should develop this internal specification and provide it to you in order to enable their compliance to the product you purchase (under contract). The most important line item developed and managed by the food safety management team in each food specification should be the microbiological specification (numbers of allowable bacteria like Total Plate Count, coliforms count, and other microorganisms found in food like yeast and mold). Chemical attributes that effect the risk for pathogen growth (e.g., pH), storage conditions required, and shelf life are also important line items within product specifications. In addition to common microbial spoilage organisms, pathogen testing can also be specified (e.g., no pathogens found after certified microbiological analysis) but should be performed as part of the HACCP plan rather than at finished product unless required by FDA/USDA or the specification includes a hold and release requirement (where the product is not released into distribution until it test negative for the designated pathogen). For example, the USDA has microbiological criteria for some foods (like eggs, ground meat) specific to pathogen hazards (like *E. coli* 0157 or *L. monocytogenes*) that a manufacturer must comply to in order to sell these foods to retail food businesses. The USDA lists several helpful references to aid in the determination of what microbiological standards should be used for foods (both to prevent spoilage, estimate shelf life, and setting microbiological standards for foods to prevent pathogen hazards) on its Food Safety Research Information Office, Microbiological Standards and Guidelines web page (USDA 2012a). The FDA and USDA also have well-established methods that should be followed to perform microbiological analysis of foods (FDA 2012a; USDA 2012b), and these standard methods should be used to provide assurance (via third party laboratories) that the microbiological data has no errors.

Because many allergic customers of retail food service establishments consume food based on knowledge of its ingredients (i.e., they usually seek this information before they consume a product if they are extremely allergic to an ingredient, e.g., peanuts), it is be important for the retail food business to ensure ingredient integrity of the products manufactured for its retail units and the means to ensure manufactures are strictly compliant to the ingredient specifications. For example,

I.	Commitment	VIII.	Document Control
a.	Management Policy		and Records
b.	Management Responsi-bility	a.	Document Control
		b.	Records
c.	Food Safety and Quality Management System	IX.	Allergen Control
d.	Management Review	a.	Allergen control program
e.	Complaint Management	b.	Control of new and/or modified product formulation
f.	Business Continuity Planning		
II.	Specification and Product Development	c.	Control at purchasing of ingredients
a.	Product Development and Realization	d.	Control of new and/or modified labels
b.	Raw Materials	e.	Control at receiving of ingredients and externally printed labels
c.	Packaging		
d.	Contract Service Providers	f.	Control at weighing, blending, mixing, formulation steps
e.	Contract Manufacturers		
f.	Finished Product	g.	Control of rework product
g.	Incoming Goods and Services		
h.	Corrective and Preventative Action	h.	Control at labeling of finished product
i.	Non-conforming Product or Equipment	i.	Control of obsolete materials Control of cross-contamination
j.	Product Rework		
k.	Product Release	X.	Verification
l.	Stock Rotation	a.	Responsibility, Frequency and Methods
III.	Product Identification		
a.	Product Trace	b.	Validation
b.	Product Withdrawal and Recall	c.	Verification of Monitoring Activities
c.	Site Security	d.	Product Sampling, Inspection and Analysis
IV.	Food Defense		
a.	Physical Security	e.	Inspections
b.	Storage	f.	Verification Schedule
		g.	Product Identification, Trace, Withdrawal and Recall

Fig. 4.4 Example prerequisite system requirements of a manufacturing facility

suppose I am allergic to peanuts, and I plan to consume a desert from a restaurant I trust based on its declared ingredients list for the product that states there are no peanuts in the product (observed at their web site or nutrition brochure). However, because the desert is manufactured for the restaurant in a facility that processes peanuts (and the restaurant company choose not to declare this on their ingredient statement to reduce avoidance of their deserts). Now suppose when I consume the desert I have an allergic reaction (possibly lethal if I don't have my Epinephrine pen with me). I would expect this company to have ensured the product was peanut free if they choose to not declare it was made in a plant with peanuts especially if there is knowledge the product is made on the same processing line as other

V.	Building and Equipment/ Design and Construction	XI.	Equipment, Utensils, cleaning, and Protective Clothing
	a. Site Requirements and Approval		a. Cleaning of Processing Equipment, Utensils and Protective Clothing
	b. Premises Location		b. Hand Washing Facilities
	c. Construction and Operational Approval		c. Protective Clothing Racks
	d. Food Handling Areas	XII.	Water and Ice Supply
	e. Materials and Surfaces		a. Water Supply
	f. Floors, Drains and Waste Traps		b. Water Delivery
	g. Walls, Partitions, Doors and Ceilings		c. Ice Supply
	h. Stairs, Catwalks and Platforms		d. Water Treatment
	i. Lighting and Light Fitings	XIII.	Storage Facilities
	j. Inspection Area		a. Cold Storage, Freezing and Chilling of Foods
	k. Dust, Fly and Vermin Proofing		b. Storage and Dry Ingredient and Other Shelf Stable Packaged Goods
	l. Ventilation		c. Storage and Packaging
VI.	Separation of Functions		d. Storage of Equipment and Receptacles
	a. Process Flow		e. Storage of Hazardous Chemicals and Toxic Substances
	b. Receipt of Raw Materials		f. Alternative Storage and Handling of Goods
	c. Thawing of Product	XIV.	Waste Disposal
	d. High Risk Processes		a. Dry and Liquid Waste Disposal.
	e. On-site Laboratories		b. Exterior
VII.	Staff Amenities		c. Grounds and Roadways
	a. General		
	b. Change Rooms		
	c. Showers		
	d. Laundry		
	e. Sanitary Facilities		
	f. Lunch Rooms		
	g. First Aid Facilities		
	h. Access to First Aid		

Fig. 4.4 (continued)

products with peanuts (requiring cleaning to remove peanut protein as a CCP). This company could have set up an undeclared allergen hold and release specification where it required the manufacture to test the ingredients and final product for peanuts to significantly reduce this risk to its customers (or declare the product may have peanuts on the ingredient list and packaging).

Many companies use data base collection software to capture all declared ingredients information for all products manufactured for the business and to enable the business to keep this information up to date for ingredient and nutrition tracking (both required to enable communication to the customer either via labeling of packaged food requirements or retail point of purchase menu brochures/web site). All packaged food products (including any packaged in the retail business) are required by the FDA/USDA to list ingredients and nutrition information on a label. Foods

Facility/capacity

- Proposed menu
- Site Plan (drawn to scale)
- Floor plan layout (drawn to scale)
- Arrangement of equipment (drawn to scale)
- Mechanical plans – plumbing (water supply/waste drain lines), HVAC (include balance equations), and lighting
- Construction materials and finish schedule
- Type and model of proposed fixed equipment and facilities
- Anticipated service volume per day

Food prep

- Garbage and refuse disposal
- Employee areas, restrooms, and hand washing sinks
- Windows, doors, and insect/rodent control
- Refrigeration and capacity
- Storage area for food and food packaging
- Sanitizing equipment and faculties
- Ware washing equipment
- Hot water supply and use (capacity)
- Laundry area
- Exhaust hood ventilation for cook line

Fig. 4.5 Example elements in a state retail plan requirement used to develop a retail prerequisite specification for a retail facility

sold by food service establishments that are prepared for immediate consumption are generally exempt from this requirement because most of the food products served to customers are packaged only for handling the food safely before purchase (i.e., this packaging has little to no ingredient information on the package nor is it required). Many chain retail food service organizations provide nutrition and ingredient information for their customers via corporate web sites and/or brochures within the retail units. In order to better align packaged food labeling requirements to that of food sold in restaurants/food service establishments (where labels are not required), new legislation (FDA 2011) will soon require nutrition information to be posted within these establishments on menu boards and other points of purchase for the customer. However, ingredient posting on menu boards or packaging will not be required.

Finished product specifications often times must also include more specific food safety procedural requirements in addition to HACCP (defined CCPs) to enable corporate control systems to be most effective like those described in the chocolate milk claim story at the beginning of this chapter. Often time, the HACCP plan is integrated into the finished product specification (which is useful to use for training employees how to make the ingredient/product), but it is better to have them identified separately as well to enable better food safety oversight of the CCPs via verification.

An important component of a finished product specification is a defined lot/batch identification process (and labeling requirement of bulk product distributed to retail units) to enable trace back and trace forward tracking of all ingredients and products manufactured for the retail food business. This enables a product traceability system (a corporate control system) to effectively limit the amount of ingredient/products effected during a recall or product withdrawal. Thus in the event of a need to recall an ingredient/product from retail sales, the food safety management team would not need to remove all such product from all retail units (if, for example, only an individual ingredient/product lot/batch were affected by a known food safety hazard) due to the ability to communicate to its retail stores to only remove the effected lot/batch from service (and stop distribution of this ingredient/product to stores). Tracking where the product was distributed to (to increase confidence in removal) and the knowledge in the safety of all other lots/batch of that ingredient/product made by the manufacturer (assuming this is verified with the manufacturer) can provide confidence in the safety of the ingredients/products in the retail units, reduce significant waste, and equip the retail units with evidence they did not serve a recalled product.

Likewise, a finished product specification, based on the nature of the product (e.g., potentially hazardous foods), should require the manufacturer to retain samples of all finished ingredients/products (labeled by lot/batch identification that includes date and time of manufacture—stored properly) until a designated time (normally the shelf life of the ingredient/product). This would speed up the ability to check microbiological and chemical safety of any defect claim on that ingredient/product, providing more confidence that the ingredient/product was safe before it entered distribution. It is not the scope of this chapter to review all of the food safety variables that might determine a final finished product specification for a manufacturer or retail unit including elements of a food safety requirement for production, but several of the most important of these are listed in Fig. 4.6 as examples (the use of each should be based on the type of ingredient/product being manufactured) because these have been useful to me to provide knowledge necessary to make good business-based public health decisions.

All retail units need a finished product specification (as part of the documented recipes) to ensure procedures are followed that will lead to effective CCP controls. The retail unit finished product specification should describe how to make and store the product including documenting all CCPs, how to check the CCPs, and corrective actions allowed in the event of CCP failure. It is likely best to integrate HACCP into the finished product specification to enable ease of food safety training of employees at the retail level. However, keeping separate HACCP plans for each product is also useful and, as mentioned above, often required by some regulatory authorities (Fig. 4.3). It should be noted that HACCP was originally designed to prevent the need for finished product testing for biological, chemical, and physical hazards. When applied appropriately, HACCP can significantly reduce cost to a retail food business (and its manufacturers) by preventing the hazard in an ingredient/product rather than discovering it and requiring destruction of the ingredient/product before it enters food distribution. HACCP is also the best foundation for a retail finished product specification for this purpose in retail units because most foods prepared in a retail environment are for immediate consumption, and thus there are no means to hold and test finished products. However, HACCP does not provide for how the product should be made but only the CCPs to check to ensure prevention of hazards.

- Shelf life of ingredient/product and storage requirements documented (e.g., best before date and temperature required to retain shelf life)
- Lot/batch identification and date/time of manufacture to enable trace back of ingredient/product (and enable location of product within distribution)
- Finished ingredient/product retained samples, testing requirements, and time required to retain samples (shelf life minimum)
- Corrective action plan for ingredient/product defects and reporting requirements
- Communications of regulatory compliance ingredient/product defects (before FDA or USDA recall or warning letter)
- Ingredient/product rework requirements (e.g., restrictions)
- Hold and release requirements if pathogen testing performed with documentation and record retention based on lot/batch and date/time of manufacture
- Additional allergen control program (undeclared allergens testing and hold and release requirements)
- Food defense plan (security based on risk assessment)
- Food quarantine plan and storage segregation of ingredient/product during na ingredient/product withdrawal or hold in distribution
- Foreign body control (e.g., x-ray/bones, metal detection/metals)requirements

Fig. 4.6 Elements of a finished product specification for ingredients/products produced by a food manufacturer

Other manufacture control systems include education specifications for retail unit employees and suppliers (discussed separately in Chap. 5) and food safety related standard operating procedures (SOPs) in both. Many SOPs in retail and supplier manufacturing facilities can control food safety hazards like cross contamination or poor personal hygiene (not washing hands properly). These SOPs should be specific to the operations and easily integrated into the flow of food prep for proper use. Cleaning and sanitation SOPs are the most common manufacture control system in retail and manufacturing facilities, but others are common like required glove use or hand washing. One example of a retail SOP is found in the FDA Food Code requirement for food handlers to wear food service gloves whenever they handle/prepare ready to eat foods (often called the No Bare Hands Contact rule). This rule if used properly can reduce risk of employees contaminating food with unclean hands often associated with poor personal hygiene (many such events are documented annually as Hepatitis A or Norovirus outbreaks in retail environments). Using color coding of gloves to differentiate handling of ready to eat foods from raw foods by employees can be used as a management tool to watch for potential cross contamination events. For example, I have used a yellow colored glove SOP requirement (when handling raw chicken) as part of the FDA's SOP on No Bare Hands Contact rule. When used correctly, employees can be trained and monitored

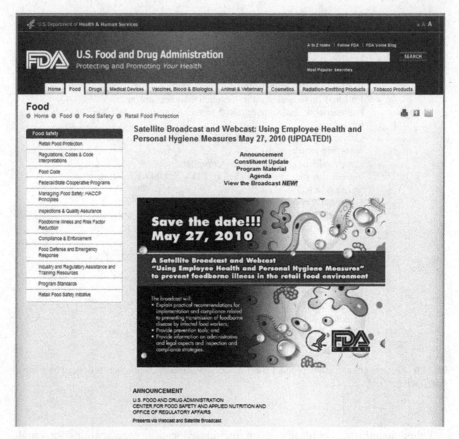

Fig. 4.7 FDA training for retail food businesses on best practices on standard operating procedures (SOPs) to meet FDA food code requirements (http://www.fda.gov/Food/FoodSafety/RetailFoodProtection/ucm211949.htm)

to ensure they do not cross contaminate food contact surfaces or ready to eat foods simply by observing proper glove use. Employees properly trained also begin to see yellow colored gloves as those that indicate their hands are contaminated with raw chicken (and possible pathogens on raw chicken) while clear gloves use is reserved for safe foods (ready to eat). More details of the effectiveness of this SOP were presented by the FDA's Satellite broadcast and webcast: Using employee health and personal hygiene measures (Fig. 4.7).

All manufacture control systems for suppliers and retail units provide a documented platform for measuring execution and verification of ingredients/products (see Chap. 7) to ensure a supplier and retail food business prepares what has been specified. These systems also then enable better ingredient/product defect investigations where you must quickly determine if the defect is due to a supplier or retail food preparation error. It is easy to see that with only two food safety manufacture control systems discussed thus far, a prerequisite system (Fig. 4.4) and a finished product specification system (Fig. 4.6), the food safety management program can more easily manage food safety of all the suppliers to the retail food business and food prep in retail units with more confidence.

Corporate Control Systems

Corporate control systems are cross functional food safety management systems that the food retail business can use to control risk that cross over several business functions in the organization e.g., a defective product that is distributed to all the retail units that requires management by several business functions (e.g., purchasing, distribution, retail units, retail operations, legal, risk management, public relations, corporate communications). Although the food safety management program may lead and initiate these systems due to its oversight of food safety in manufacturing by suppliers and retail units, their possible impact on all the business functions (e.g., replacement product available to protect sales) drives a need for joint management. Table 4.1 shows example corporate control systems that should be developed and managed by the food safety management program. A corporate control system may be used to coordinate several manufacture control systems. For example, supplier certification and verification may be performed and documented annually (and for all new suppliers) based on review and verification of prerequisite and finished product specifications.

The most important corporate control system that can have the largest impact on all business functions (e.g., cost to the business if not available or if used improperly) is the ingredient/product withdrawal/recall system. An ingredient/product withdrawal is normally performed due to quality defects rather than food safety hazards. However, whenever a food retail business is aware of a ingredient/product hazard or a supplier recall (normally voluntarily initiated by the supplier, but sometimes initiated by the USDA or FDA), it has an obligation to notify its retail units of this recall (to enable removal of the ingredient/product from service to customers), and help to ensure the ingredient/product is not distributed further to these units and not sold or given away at retail. Many food retail businesses also self-monitor their supply chain for product defects (discussed below) and perform internal ingredient/product withdrawal or recalls (due to risk) without FDA/USDA involvement to initiate. The majority of these are due to quality defects (withdrawals) or cautionary actions due to potential food safety concerns of related ingredients manufactured in a facility that has another product under a recall due to a food safety hazard. For example, if a fresh cut lettuce brand is under an FDA recall because the FDA found *L. monocytogenes* contamination in the facility that processes this lettuce, a food retail business may reject other product from this facility and/or recall product made in this facility as a precautionary measure to avoid this potential hazard (including claims made by customers who may consume product identified as being produced in this facility by the manufacturer).

At its core, a product withdrawal/recall system in a food retail business should consist of an urgent communications and compliance program (normally a phone-based interactive voice/response system that will call all retail units, deliver the withdrawal/recall message, and capture compliance in the form of reports of effected lot/batch presence/absence from all units). There are several companies that provide these services for a fee (contract) that can communicate a withdrawal/recall notice via phone, text, email to thousands of units across the United States within 2–4 h. The food safety supply chain manager normally initiates ingredient/product recalls, tracks the progress of the recall communications, and works closely with the purchasing and distribution business functions to ensure it is removed from service to customers and replacement ingredient/product is provided.

The importance of manufacture control systems (Table 4.1) and verification of these systems (and the selection of the food safety management team member responsible for this decision) is augmented here especially if there are no secondary suppliers for a withdrawn/recalled ingredient/product. This is because this action will result in lost sales until the ingredient/product can be replaced in the retail units. Thus it is better to prevent the majority of the product defects before distribution to retail units. No supplier to a retail food business desires to be a part of a withdrawal/recall and thus should work closely with the food safety management team to prevent them by use of the specified manufacture control systems. When there is a proven ingredient/product defect from a manufacturer that must be withdrawn/recalled from retail units, then the supplier is likely the responsible party and should pay for cost related to this action including cost of product, lost sales, and cost of the urgent communication program.

A second important corporate control system the food safety management team should manage is a product defect surveillance system. Surveillance is commonly used by public health organizations (see Chap. 3) to monitor public health and quickly act on possible outbreaks of foodborne illnesses. The CDC performs surveillance of laboratory confirmed cases of illness nationally (those required to be reported to the CDC in all states) as a means to quickly act to investigate the source and root cause in order to prevent additional cases of an illness. A food retail business should do the same for its suppliers and retail units as a means to measure risk and identify areas where the food safety management team can quickly act to investigate risk within its supply chain. A surveillance system designed to discover ingredient/product defects in a retail food business is thus a means to prevent foodborne illnesses as well. A supply chain-based surveillance system (one of the corporate control systems, see Table 4.1) not only functions to detect ingredient/product defects before they become a hazard at the retail level, but can reduce significant cost to the business the earlier the defect is detected (including if you prevent the cost of product withdrawals/recalls). A supply chain-based surveillance system should actually be composed of several independent reporting components (Fig. 4.8) that function to detect and report on defects at both the retail level and the supply level, and of which enable the food safety management team to take action based on real-time information.

First, the team should set up automatic e-alerts from the FDA and USDA for all regulatory actions related to food suppliers. For example, the FDA has a web site .

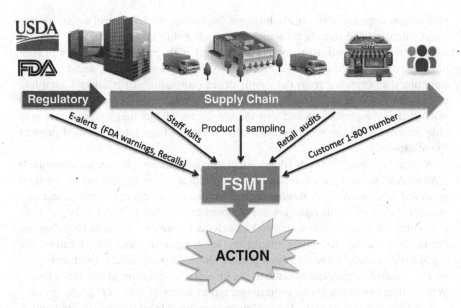

Fig. 4.8 A supply chain-based surveillance system to detect ingredient/product defects; monitored by the food safety management team (FSMT)

that reports all monthly actions related to its enforcement (called the FDA warning letters) that includes actions taken with food manufactures related to food safety issues discover during FDA sponsored facilities and/or product audits (FDA 2012c). These e-alerts are emails sent from the FDA that provide notice of food manufactures (listed by company name) that have been given warning by the FDA due to food safety hazards identified in their faculties. This information enables regulatory compliance surveillance of the businesses suppliers wherein the food safety management team can investigate and take action (e.g., initiate third-party audit, visit from staff, withdrawal of products, or removing the facility from the approved ingredients/products suppliers to the business).

The second important surveillance date the team can collect is via e-alerts of FDA/USDA recalls (see Foodsafety.gov 2012). These emails can be easily monitored by the food safety management team based on keyword notice (e.g., using email software programs that highlight specific emails with their supplier's brand names/products). Some companies also provide e-alert services augmented by media report surveillance of your company's brand name as a key word. Google Alerts (which is free) can also monitor the internet for any mention of company specific key words including association with recalls and/or FDA/USDA actions. These surveillance tools can augment the visibility of the risk within a supply chain (from manufacturers to retail units).

Other important information that can be used within a product defect surveillance system in the supply chain include physical data normally collected via the verification responsibilities of the business (including quality control verifications). Food safety related data (e.g., temperatures, shelf-life compliance, SOP compliance) in reports from third-party and food safety management team audits of supplier and retail facilities can be captured by facility and product name. Product sampling data captured from the supply chain (normally quality control sampling to measure weights, piece counts, etc. but can include temperature of product etc.) at both the manufacturing and distribution levels of the supply chain can provide information to be monitored for compliance to food safety finished product specifications.

A retail unit level reporting tool that can also support surveillance for ingredient/product defects can be used to screen for and capture some defects before the food is served to customers. A routine ingredient/product receiving, storing, and raw product evaluation at the retail level and means to report these data can be essential in capturing common ingredient/product defects before they become larger issues. Product evaluation procedures should include a reporting tool (retail audits; see Fig. 4.8) that enables retail units to report ingredient/product defects (and seek credits for defective ingredients/products; an incentive to perform at the retail level). When a data base system can capture and report identical defects (e.g., by product type, lot/batch number) to the food safety management team (across all retail units), the team can then investigate and make better food safety decisions. These data can also be used to make decisions on internal product withdrawals/recalls but are most commonly used for product withdrawals based on quality not food safety defects. Nevertheless, this retail audit supply chain-based surveillance enables early prevention of larger number of customers receiving a food safety hazard in a ready to eat food when this system is monitored carefully and then used with the product withdrawal/recall communication and compliance system.

Finally, the last and most common process used to capture retail product defects is the customer complaint program (e.g., 1–800 number for customers to call with their complaints about a product/service). A recent study by Li et al. (2011) found that complaint rates of customers was positively correlated to foodborne disease outbreaks with 69% of outbreaks detected through customer complaints to local health departments. In other words, when customers complain and more than one complains about the same food, it may be a leading indicator of a current food safety issue in that retail unit. This can be an effective tool for food safety surveillance (and is used most often for quality-related issues effectively) if the information is monitored, investigated, and acted upon by the food safety management team in real time. For example, if a customer called the 1–800 customer complaint line or emailed about a food safety complaint (e.g., feeling sick after drinking a packaged chocolate milk product), and these complaints were delivered (via voice mail or email) to a designated food safety management team member who monitors and investigates these claims, they could determine the validity of the claim (as demonstrated in the scenario at the beginning of the chapter including additional review of probability based on verified effective manufacture control systems), and possibly prevent additional illnesses (if confirmed) by initiating a recall.

Over time, continual monitoring and system evaluations collectively enable the food safety management team to determine the likely root cause of most ingredient/product defects. Some defects may be due to manufacture error at the retail level of which all customer complaints would be linked to that one retail unit. Of course, surveillance of customer food safety complaints must be rigorously monitored and investigated, or it can lead to increased liability to the business when food safety data is collected but not investigated. Therefore, a redundant system should be in place that includes a requirement for the retail operator to also investigate and follow up with all food safety complaints by customers in addition to members of the food safety management team.

It is not feasible to list and discuss all systems necessary to ensure control of food safety hazards within a food retail business here. Many of the systems described may not always fit each retail business due to scale of the business, and there are others that have not been described that may be equally important to control hazards (e.g., Six Sigma quality control programs for manufactures) within specific retail food business operations. However, the systems discussed in this chapter should serve as a foundation that the food safety management program should have in place as the minimum requirements to manage food safety hazards within the business.

References

Brown M, Stringer M (2002) Microbiological risk assessment in food processing. CRC Press LLC, Boca Raton, FL

CAC (Codex Alimentarius Commission) (1997) Hazard analysis and critical control point system and guidelines for its application. Annex to CAC/RCP 1-1969, Rev. 3-1997. Rome: Food and agriculture Organization of the United Nations

CFR, Title 21, Part 110 (2011) Available via the internet at http://www.accessdata.fda.gov/scripts/cdrh/cfdocs/cfcfr/CFRSearch.cfm?CFRPart=110&showFR=1

FDA (1997) Hazard analysis and critical control point principles and application guidelines. Available via the internet at http://www.fda.gov/food/foodsafety/HazardAnalysisCriticalControlPointsHACCP/ucm114868.htm

FDA (2006) Managing food safety: a manual for voluntary use of HACCP principles for operators of food service and retail establishments. Available via the internet at http://www.fda.gov/downloads/Food/FoodSafety/RetailFoodProtection/ManagingFoodSafetyHACCPPrinciples/Operators/UCM077957.pdf

FDA (2009a) Food code, Annex4-Management of food safety practices–Achieving active managerial control of foodborne illness risk factors

FDA (2009b) Analysis and evaluation of preventive control measures for the control and reduction/elimination of microbial hazards on fresh and fresh-cut produce, chapter V, methods to reduce/eliminate pathogens from produce and fresh-cut produce. Available via internet at http://www.fda.gov/Food/ScienceResearch/ResearchAreas/SafePracticesforFoodProcesses/ucm091363.htm

FDA (2011) New menu and vending machines labeling requirements. Available via the internet at http://www.fda.gov/Food/LabelingNutrition/ucm217762.htm

FDA (2012a) Bacteriological analytical manual (BAM). Available via the internet at http://www.fda.gov/Food/ScienceResearch/LaboratoryMethods/BacteriologicalAnalyticalManualBAM/default.htm

FDA (2012b) The new FDA food safety modernization act (FSMA). Available via the internet at http://www.fda.gov/food/foodsafety/fsma/default.htm

FDA (2012c) Inspections, compliance, enforcement, and criminal investigations. Available via the internet at http://www.fda.gov/ICECI/EnforcementActions/WarningLetters/default.htm

Fishburn J et al (2012) Efficacy of various consumer-friendly produce washing technologies in reducing pathogens on fresh produce. Food Protect Trends 32:456–466

Foodsafety.gov. (2012) Get automatic alerts. Available via internet at http://www.foodsafety.gov/recalls/alerts/index.html

FSIS (1996) Pathogen reduction: hazard analysis and critical control point (HACCP) systems; Final rule. Fed Regist 61:38805–38855

Institute of Medicine, National Research Council (2003) Scientific criteria to ensure safe food. The National Academies Press, Washington, DC

Li J et al (2011) Complaint-based surveillance for foodborne illness in the United States: a survey of local health departments. J Food Prot 74:432–437

Maryland Department of Health and Mental Hygiene (2008) Guidelines for submitting a hazard analysis critical control point (HACCP) plan. Available via the internet at http://ideha.dhmh.maryland.gov/OEHFP/OFPCHS/Shared%20Documents/plan-review/guidelines/HACCP%20Guidelines_Nov2008ver.pdf

Panglol PHY, Beuchat LR, King CH, Zhao Z (2009) Reduction of *Escherichia coli* O157:H7 on produce by use of electrolyzed water under simulated food service operation conditions. J Food Prot 72:1854–1861

Parish ME, Beuchat LR, Suslow TV, Haris LJ, Garret EH, Farber JN, Busta FF (2003) Methods to reduce/eliminate pathogens from fresh and fresh-cut produce, chap. 5. In Analysis and evaluation of preventive control measure for the control and reduction/elimination of microbial hazards on fresh and fresh-cut produce. Comp Rev Food Sci Food Saf 2(Suppl):161–173

Stevenson KE, Bernard DT (1995) HACCP, establishing hazard analysis critical control point programs. A workshop manual, 2nd edn. Food Processors Institute, Washington, DC

USDA (2012) Microbiology laboratory guidebook. Available via the internet at http://www.fsis.usda.gov/science/microbiological_lab_guidebook/

USDA (2012a) Microbiological standards and guidelines. Available via the internet at http://fsrio.nal.usda.gov/sanitation-and-quality-standards/microbiological-standards-and-guidelines

Chapter 5
Education and Training

Education is what you achieve after training. In the retail food business, it should be defined purposely based on what you want others not usually educated in food safety to know and do. In order for an employee to sustain an education (and thus competency to perform task and own food safety responsibility), there must be a formal training process targeted to the required knowledge. There should also be a structured curriculum based on the prerequisite experience of the employee, food safety specifications built into the task (e.g., recipes), a means to deliver the training to diverse students (e.g., age, language, lack of food service experience), hands-on demonstration, and a method to measure education of the student via knowledge test and application of the knowledge. The food safety training must also be appropriate to the education needed (and level of comprehension of the employee) at each position of food_safety management desired at the retail level (food handler vs. manager) and corporate staff level, and required for all employees. Finally, the same curriculum should be offered in different delivery methods that will accommodate the students' best means to learn and demonstrate competency (e.g., online Spanish course vs. lecture), and food safety education should be validated on a regular basis (audited) to determine when additional training is necessary.

Levels of Training in a Food Retail Business

A retail food business has multiple positions where employees may need to know basic to advanced levels of food safety knowledge within its retail units, within its business functions, and within its supplier facilities. All of the food safety training materials must be built upon a foundation of regulatory requirements and manufacture control systems specific to each. For example, all education within a supplier's facilities (not normally a function of a retail food business to provide but must be verified) is expected to ensure employees are trained to prevent hazards during production of ingredients/products supplied to the retail business. Basing all food safety education on HACCP and GFSI systems and specifications training

H. King, *Food Safety Management: Implementing a Food Safety Program in a Food Retail Business*, Food Microbiology and Food Safety, DOI 10.1007/978-1-4614-6205-7_5, © Springer Science+Business Media New York 2013

requirements ensures that all business partners, their employees, and staff in various business functions that manage supplier relationships are trained to the same food safety standards. Likewise, when all retail food units are trained on FDA Food Code-specified food safety training expectations (and all food preparation procedures are based on the same, e.g., no bare hands contact allowed with ready-to-eat food prep), an accepted standard is established that all business functions (e.g., training department, field operations department) can follow. These standards then allow for uniform delivery of the training materials and verification of training (i.e., was there education as evidenced by application of the requirements) throughout the supply chain.

Suppliers

The successful implementation and verification of any manufacture control system (including but most importantly HACCP) is the training program that ensures competency and compliance to requirements. A HACCP program requires (and should be visible in all training materials) that each employee (line level to manager) is educated in the principles of HACCP, how to identify hazards (important even to line-level employees so they can recognize similar hazards that may arise due to changes in production), and how to implement proper controls. Most importantly, each employee must know how to monitor each CCP and make appropriate corrective actions when a CCP fails to ensure hazard prevention. Each employee must also be trained on the tools necessary to monitor CPs and CCPs. If a food safety management program has limited resources to comprehensively verify food safety within the facilities of its suppliers, requiring HACCP program verification data with evidence of this training would be one of the most cost-effective means for hazard prevention. Because HACCP is part of GMPs and soon to be enforced by the FDA/USDA via authority of FSMA (where hazard identification and prevention systems must be documented), alignment to HACCP helps to ensure a food retail business is purchasing its ingredients/products from suppliers that meet or exceed regulatory requirements.

Within any prerequisite specification (a manufacture control system), a manufacturer manages multiple business functions (see Fig. 4.4) that require specific training in each area, for example, cleaning and sanitation of processing equipment or pest control, each critical to the safe production of food (undeclared allergen prevention or prevention of pest infestations of the facilities). Although it is not the function of a retail business to determine and verify the training and education to each of these elements, requiring a third-party certification, industry-benchmarked food safety standard like GFSI scheme (one that performs annual audits to document a manufacturers commitment to education) validates proper training specifications are in place. It is also a more cost-effective means to verify (via additional audits) that proper training is being performed to educate employees to prevent defined hazards in their facilities during production of ingredients/products.

Retail Units

As with the supplier-level manufacture training alignment to regulatory requirements (FDA/USDA), all retail unit training should also be aligned to the FDA Food Code (FDA 2012b) and HACCP. This is even more critical in the retail food service establishments of the business because the majority of local and state regulators enforce food safety rules based on the FDA Food Code via local inspections (and communicate risk based inspection scoring/grading of the units to the public). It is best to ensure all food prep and food safety requirements in all units align to the most current FDA Food Code especially if the food retail units are located in multiple states. This then ensures that all units uniformly follow the best science in prevention of foodborne illnesses, and training of employees on this one standard will ensure regulators can easily inspect and observe food safety compliance (see Chap. 10 to learn more about how this helps the food retail business partner with public health officials) to food code requirements in their jurisdiction.

More importantly, each employee should be trained on how the business complies to key FDA Food Code rules in order to educate them to work with health inspectors who are tasked to verify compliance for public health. For example, suppose your method to keep ready-to-eat (RTE) foods out of the temperature danger zone (41°F–135 °F) is based on temperature (e.g., you maintain all hot hold products throughout the day above 135 °F) rather than time (you do not track time nor allow RTE foods to be stored below this temperature at any time). When the local health inspector visits one of your retail units, it scores a violation expecting to see the establishment track time for each RTE food, if the employees are not trained on the methods the retail establishment uses to comply to this rule, so the inspector requires the RTE food to be discarded (a significant food cost loss if this occurs often). The FDA Food Code rule (RTE hot foods must be maintained at 135 °F or above at all times or if held under this temperature, must be tracked for time and discarded after more than 4 h maximum time) allows you to use one or the other method to keep RTE foods out of the temperature danger zone (see Fig. 5.1). If the employees have this education, they will be able to demonstrate that the retail establishment is allowed to hold the food throughout the day at 135 °F or above without tracking time (and most likely sales the food well before 1–2 h due to quality need).

All managers (and of course the owner/operator) of all retail units should be trained to the minimum level of food safety education via a Certified Food Safety Manager (CFSM) course or other American National Standards Institute (ANSI) food safety certification standard (e.g., by certification bodies like National Restaurant Association's ServSafe, Prometric's Certified Professional Food Manager (CPFM), or National Environmental Health Association's Certified Professional in Food Safety (CP-FS)) course. This curriculum standard (although slightly different in how is it structured and taught by each certification body) is aligned to the most current FDA Food Code (and is accredited by the FDA through this standard), teaches managers the principles of food safety hazard identification, and teaches the standard methods to prevent these known hazards.

3-501.16 Potentially Hazardous Food (Time/Temperature Control for Safety Food), Hot and Cold Holding.

1. (A) *Except during preparation, cooking, or cooling, or when time is used as the public health control as specified under §3-501.19,* and except as specified under ¶ (B) and in ¶ (C) of this section, POTENTIALLY HAZARDOUS FOOD (TIME/TEMPERATURE CONTROL FOR SAFETY FOOD) shall be maintained:

    (1) At 57°C (135°F) or above, *except that roasts cooked to a temperature and for a time specified in ¶ 3-401.11(B) or reheated as specified in ¶ 3-403.11(E) may be held at a temperature of 54°C (130°F) or above;* [P] or

    (2) At 5°C (41°F) or less. [P]

2. (B) EGGS that have not been treated to destroy all viable *Salmonellae* shall be stored in refrigerated EQUIPMENT that maintains an ambient air temperature of 7°C (45°F) or less. [P]

3. (C) POTENTIALLY HAZARDOUS FOOD (TIME/TEMPERATURE CONTROL FOR SAFETY FOOD) in a homogenous liquid form *may be maintained outside of the temperature control requirements, as specified under ¶ (A) of this section, while contained within specially designed EQUIPMENT that complies with the design and construction requirements as specified under ¶ 4-204.13(E).*

OR

3-501.19 Time as a Public Health Control.

1. (A) Except as specified under ¶ (D) of this section, if time without temperature control is used as the public health control for a working supply of POTENTIALLY HAZARDOUS FOOD (TIME/TEMPERATURE CONTROL FOR SAFETY FOOD) before cooking, or for READY-TO-EAT POTENTIALLY HAZARDOUS FOOD (TIME/TEMPERATURE CONTROL FOR SAFETY FOOD) that is displayed or held for sale or service:

    1. (1) Written procedures shall be prepared in advance, maintained in the FOOD ESTABLISHMENT and made available to the REGULATORY AUTHORITY upon request that specify: [Pf]

        1. (a) Methods of compliance with Subparagraphs (B)(1)-(3) or C)(1)-(5) of this section; [Pf] and
        2. (b) Methods of compliance with § 3-501.14 for FOOD that is prepared, cooked, and refrigerated before time is used as a public health control. [Pf]

    (B) If time temperature control is used as the public health control up to a maximum of 4 hours:

    (1) The FOOD shall have an initial temperature of 5°C (41°F) or less when removed from cold holding temperature control, or 57°C (135°F) or greater when removed from hot holding temperature control; [P]

    (2) The FOOD shall be marked or otherwise identified to indicate the time that is 4 hours past the point in time when the FOOD is removed from temperature control; [Pf]

    (3) The FOOD shall be cooked and served, served at any temperature if READY-TO-EAT, or discarded, within 4 hours from the point in time when the FOOD is removed from temperature control; [P] and

    (4) The FOOD in unmarked containers or PACKAGES, or marked to exceed a 4-hour limit shall be discarded. [P]

Fig. 5.1 FDA Food Code rules on time and temperature control for retail food service establishments (FDA 2012b)

In 2006, the CDC endorsed the presence of a CFSM in food service establishments, stating that having a CFSM (performing active managerial control of food safety hazards) on-site during all operations of a food service establishment is one of the more important means to prevent a foodborne illness outbreak from a retail establishment (CDC 2006). This endorsement was based on a CDC-funded study (Hedberg et al. 2006) that showed that the most significant difference between restaurants that were associated with foodborne disease outbreaks was the presence of a CFSM, which were also associated with compliance to no bare hands contact with foods. This report and CDC's endorsement suggest that the education of the person in charge within a retail food establishment has a direct influence on the behaviors of the employees handling foods and correlates directly to public health.

Many states require that a retail food business unit have a CFSM as the owner/operator of the business, and some retail food businesses require that a CFSM is on-site during all operation of a retail unit. Because the certification course developed by these ANSI certification bodies does not teach specific application of these principles in the systems and specifications (e.g., food safety SOPs) of specific (e.g., Chick-fil-A) a retail unit's menu (which is important to do in order to ensure a manufacture control system like HACCP), an additional training necessary after this certification for all managers should be the specific active managerial control food safety training course specific to the retail businesses menu and food prep procedures. The components of this training should be based on the ingredients and foods produced and facilities' design in each retail establishment but should also include all the components defined in Fig. 5.2 (FDA Food Code recommendations for the education a manager should have to enable active managerial control). The Certified Food Safety Manager (CFSM) courses do teach many of these elements, but many of the applications are general to retail businesses (e.g., storage of food, cooking, etc.) and more specific recipe based HACCP should form the basis of additional manager training to ensure active managerial control. Additionally, development of an advanced food safety management training that integrates methods of verification (see Chap. 7) and how to perform corrective actions (especially for CCPs) is important as the final means to ensure active managerial control education includes prevention of food safety hazards. Once managers are empowered with this education, they will be able to more capably train other employees as well.

A food handler (sometimes called employee level or non-manager level) food safety course is offered by several of the same ANSI-accredited certification bodies above (and others). However, it is better that a food retail business establish its own food safety employee requirements (e.g., health policy, personal hygiene, etc.) and develop training materials and evaluations based on this to align best with its own food prep specifications/recipes (an example of a curriculum standard for a food handler education requirement in retail establishments that handle raw and RTE foods is shown in Fig. 5.3). Many of the retail units systems (e.g., food safety SOPs) and specifications should be integrated into the food handler curriculum to ensure food handlers can follow all requirements properly. Each employee should demonstrate food safety education via curriculum-based exams (oral or written are best) and demonstrate the important food safety SOPs via application during work

(D) How can the occurrence of foodborne illness risk factors be reduced?

To effectively reduce the occurrence of foodborne illness risk factors, operators of retail and food service establishments must focus their efforts on achieving active managerial control . The term "active managerial control" is used to describe industry's responsibility for developing and implementing food safety management systems to prevent, eliminate, or reduce the occurrence of foodborne illness risk factors.

Active managerial control means the purposeful incorporation of specific actions or procedures by industry management into the operation of their business to attain control over foodborne illness risk factors. It embodies a preventive rather than reactive approach to food safety through a continuous system of monitoring and verification.

There are many tools that can be used by industry to provide active managerial control of foodborne illness risk factors. Regulatory inspections and follow-up activities must also be proactive by using an inspection process designed to assess the degree of active managerial control that retail and food service operators have over the foodborne illness risk factors. In addition, regulators must assist operators in developing and implementing voluntary strategies to strengthen existing industry systems to prevent the occurrence of foodborne illness risk factors. Elements of an effective food safety management system may include the following:

o Certified food protection managers who have shown a proficiency in required information by passing a test that is part of an accredited program
o Standard operating procedures (SOPs) for performing critical operational steps in a food preparation process, such as cooling
o Recipe cards that contain the specific steps for preparing a food item and the food safety critical limits, such as final cooking temperatures, that need to be monitored and verified
o Purchase specifications
o Equipment and facility design and maintenance
o Monitoring procedures
o Record keeping
o Employee health policy for restricting or excluding ill employees
o Manager and employee training
o On-going quality control and assurance
o Specific goal-oriented plans, like Risk Control Plans (RCPs), that outline procedures for controlling foodborne illness risk factors.

Fig. 5.2 Other elements of a retail food manager's food safety education to enable active managerial control of food safety management systems to prevent, eliminate, or reduce the occurrence of foodborne illness risk factors (from FDA 2012a, b)

(e.g., hand washing and proper glove use) overseen by the CFSM. Most important to this education is the awareness of when not to work when the employee has an illness (normally taught in personal hygiene training but should be emphasized as dealing with an illness) that could lead to a food safety hazard in the establishment brought in by the employee.

Many foodborne disease outbreaks (too numerous to cite here) are associated with employees who work and handle food while sick with a foodborne illness (or a disease that is also acquired from other sources but is also spread by food, e.g., norovirus infections). For example, a food handler infected with norovirus (and in a contagious phase) that does not wash hands properly and/or wear food service gloves can infect a significant number of customers (sometimes only limited by the number of foods the employee handles). The FDA has an excellent resource (called

I.   Importance of Food Safety
II.   Contamination Hazards and Prevention
        a.   Biological/Microbial Contamination of Food
        b.   Physical Contamination of Food
        c.   Chemical Contamination of Food
        d.   Cross-Contamination
        e.   Critical Control Points (CCPs)
III.   Personal Hygiene and Health
        a.   Washing and Sanitizing Hands
        b.   Wearing Gloves
        c.   Dealing with Illness
        d.   Dealing with Injury or Infection on Hands
        e.   Grooming, Uniforms and Food Safety
        f.   Eating at Work
IV.   Controlling Temperature and Time
        a.   Temperature Danger Zone
        b.   Breaking Bacterial Growth Cycle
        c.   Keeping Cold Food Safe
        d.   Keeping Hot Food Safe
        e.   Checking Product Temperatures
        f.   Maintaining Thermometers
V.   Receiving and Storing Food Safely
        a.   Approved Suppliers and Produce Brands
        b.   Receiving Food Safely
        c.   Storing Food Safely
VI.   Cleaning and Sanitizing
        a.   Preparing and Maintaining Sanitizing Solution
        b.   Cleaning and Sanitizing Food Contact Surfaces
        c.   Cleaning and Maintaining Towels Safely
        d.   Cleaning Floors Safely
        e.   Cleaning Up Body Fluids Safely
        f.   Handling Trash Safely
VII.   Preparing Produce Safely
VIII.   Preparing Raw Foods Safely
IX.   Preparing and Cooking Food Safely
X.   Serving Food and Beverages Safely
        a.   Ice handling safety
XI.   Food Allergies and Intolerance
        a.   Things You Need to Know
        b.   Common Allergenic Products
        c.   Avoiding Cross-Contamination of Allergens and Other
              Substances
        d.   Answering Questions about Allergens
        e.   Appropriate Responses.

Fig. 5.3 Example criteria for food-handler-level employee food safety certification (education) in a retail food service establishment that handles raw and RTE foods

the *Retail Food Protection: Employee Health and Personal Hygiene Handbook* ; see FDA 2010) that can serve as the foundation of a retail food businesses education program to train both the food handler and manager on how to prevent these types of foodborne disease outbreaks. This resource should be integrated into the education curriculum for both types of employees (managers and non managers). Many states require evidence (as part of their state food code rules) of this training as well, often called a health policy or employee personal hygiene training.

Another important education all employees should have to prevent a foodborne disease outbreak should be a body fluid cleaning and sanitation SOP. Once a customer or employee produces body fluids in a retail environment, pathogens in the body fluid can quickly contaminate food contact surfaces leading to cross contamination of foods even if the employee wears food service gloves (i.e., practices no bare hands contact with RTE foods). Many of the pathogens are also more resistant to common food service sanitizers (e.g., norovirus), making it even more important to both exclude sick employees from handling food and being prepared to clean up body fluids safely. A classic example of a foodborne disease outbreak caused by an employee's body fluid was reported in a Morbidity and Mortality Weekly Report (MMWR) by CDC (CDC 2007). A food service employee who vomited inside a restaurant where he worked caused over 364 customers to get sick with norovirus even though the employee vomited into a trash can in the kitchen and did not work with food after this illness. The CDC stated that in order to prevent this type of outbreak, "The findings underscore the need for (1) *ongoing education* of food-service workers regarding prevention of norovirus contamination and transmission; (2) enforcement of policies regarding ill and recently ill food-service workers; and (3) environmental decontamination with effective disinfectants to eliminate the presence of norovirus." (CDC 2007). Having a body fluid cleaning SOP and training all employees on this SOP (one that disinfects norovirus and other pathogens) would be an important insurance in preventing this food safety hazard. Several food safety-centered businesses sell body fluid cleanup kits that are allowed by FDA to be used in a food service establishment.

Some states, for example, California and Florida (see California Restaurant Association 2012), require a food handler certification training of all food employees working within a food service establishment. Inspectors require evidence of this training either via a card (like a license to prepare food safely). In some cases, violation of this requirement can lead to fines up to $1,000 or closure of the retail unit until training requirements are met. The primary reason why states like Florida or California establish these public health laws is because some retail food service establishments don't often train their employees on food safety requirements to prevent a foodborne illness (e.g., not working while with a Hepatitis A infection). Clearly, by developing internal training curriculum based on the food prep procedures/recipes of a retail food business and FDA Food Code, the business will be prepared to meet local and state food safety training requirements (and likely be accepted in less of an additional food handler course) and ensure food safety is managed properly within its retail units.

Training Tools

A critical aspect of training is the tools used to document, deliver, and evaluate the training has archived food safety education. Many food retail businesses focus on "hands-on" and/or "word-of-mouth" training because of labor cost concerns and/or time restraints. However, without a standard to train to, there can really be no food safety education because employees will gravitate to what is easiest to get work done. It is important that the food retail business documents its entire current training curriculum (for food handler employees and managers described above) to provide the foundation of expected employee education to work in the retail units. However, it is equally important to document (as discussed above) both the training and when the training occurred in order to show regulatory compliance and for cases where evidence is needed in support for management actions that might also result in termination of employment.

Although language-specific paper-based training materials are fine if augmented with training videos in the common language of the employee, many retail businesses are also using tablet-based computers (which bundle written SOPs, video, and exams including hands-on observations) and online training tools to enable employee food safety training. These tools also enable training verification to be linked to other verifications of food safety requirements where improper behaviors (e.g., lack of training or comprehension) may be noted during the verification process and retraining of an employee assigned as a corrective action.

In order to sustain the most current food safety education (ownership of food safety responsibilities at all levels of the organization) within the continually changing environment that occurs in a food retail unit, there must be tools in place to enable continuous updates to the training curriculum (that is required to ensure food safety education of retail employees) on a regular basis defined by risk (e.g., updated as menu changes and/or regulatory requirements change, see Chaps. 7 and 8). There should also be a regular schedule (you might call this education maintenance) of training for all employees including managers based on how long the employee works within the retail unit. For example, most managers should be trained in a CFSM course every 3 years (most states require this time frame for recertification if they require a CFSM). Food handler employees should be trained before they start working in the retail unit and then retrained on a periodic schedule based on the changes in menu and facilities of the retail units or when specific new food safety SOPs are established based on new systems or specifications initiated in the business.

Corporate Level Training and Education

As discussed in Chap. 2, each member of the food safety management team should already have competency in food safety or food science in order to perform their management responsibilities. However, if not, the business will benefit from better decisions by these team members if it supports this minimum education (food science, food safety, epidemiology, microbiology degrees) of each member on the food safety management team. Additional training in project management (if the team members do not have advanced degrees) is recommended, but this education can be acquired through experience in leading projects (initiating new work and implementing a rollout). All corporate staff that work directly in the supplier and retail business functions of the organization should also have a minimum food safety education at the level of a certified food safety manager (CFSM discussed above). This is especially important for all retail business field staff that work with the retail unit operators/managers. It is best that they receive this training alongside the owners/managers to foster partnerships in food safety management and ownership of this responsibility for the food retail business.

References

California Restaurant Association (2012) California Food Handler Card, SB 602 requires workers to receive food safety training. Available via internet at http://www.calrest.org/issues-policies/key-issues/food-safety/foodhandler/

CDC (2006) CDC Endorses Certification of Food Safety Kitchen Managers. Available via internet at http://www.cdc.gov/nceh/ehs/EHSNet/resources/certification.htm

CDC (2007) Norovirus outbreak associated with Ill food-service workers, Michigan, January–February 2006. MMWR 56(46):1212–1216. Also available via internet at http://www.cdc.gov/mmwr/preview/mmwrhtml/mm5646a2.htm

FDA (2010) Retail food protection: employee health and personal hygiene handbook. Available via internet at http://www.fda.gov/downloads/Food/FoodSafety/RetailFoodProtection/IndustryandRegulatoryAssistanceandTrainingResources/UCM194575.pdf

FDA (2012a) Food Code 2009: Annex 4 - Management of Food Safety Practices – Achieving Active Managerial Control of Foodborne Illness Risk Factors. Available via internet at http://www.fda.gov/Food/FoodSafety/RetailFoodProtection/FoodCode/FoodCode2009/ucm188363.htm

FDA (2012b) Food Code 2009. Available via internet at http://www.fda.gov/Food/FoodSafety/RetailFoodProtection/FoodCode/FoodCode2009/default.htm

Hedberg C et al (2006) Systematic environmental evaluations to identify food safety differences between outbreak and nonoutbreak restaurants. J Food Prot 69:2697–2702

Chapter 6
Facilities and Capabilities

A key business function of a food retail business is the development of the design and construction specifications of its retail units. These specifications should be documented and managed within the design and construction business function/department simply because they likely change often due to cost (e.g., real estate, construction materials), menu changes, local regulatory requirements (building codes), and interior design needs of the companies' brands. These designs should be based on food establishment plan review requirements of the FDA and individual state food codes (which define the food safety specifications for equipment and facility design) and ensure they include expected flow of food (from receiving to point of purchase), food preparation/separation, and storage needs specific to the retail food establishment's menu. Equipment should be certified to safely cook, hold, prepare, and cool foods, and equipment placement should be a critical design in the flow of food within the facility. Another business function that is often assumed to be only a supplier responsibility is the design and flow of food in a food suppliers manufacturing facility to ensure the capacity and cleaning/sanitation requirements for the safe production of ingredients and products. This includes assurance of each facility's food defense/security to ensure food under its control will not be subject to tampering or other criminal, or terrorist actions.

Retail Food Establishment Facilities

The two most definitive resources to design a retail unit plan to enable the safe production of food (and ensure regulatory compliance) are the FDA Food Establishment Plan Review Guide—produced by the FDA *and* Conference for Food Protection (FDA 2000)—and the local or state plan review guidelines (which local building codes likely require and will be regulated by the local environmental health authorities, i.e., health department). Generally, a food safety-based plan review guideline will include food safety-based requirements (i.e., definitions defined in the FDA and state food codes) to show flow of food based on the menu, facilities to maintain

H. King, *Food Safety Management: Implementing a Food Safety Program in a Food Retail Business*, Food Microbiology and Food Safety, DOI 10.1007/978-1-4614-6205-7_6,
© Springer Science+Business Media New York 2013

product temperature and to protect food, hand washing and ware washing facilities, water supply and sewage disposal (and plumbing/cross-connections), hot water capacity, food equipment and installation (location), dry storage, floors, walls, ceiling finish, restroom design/location, lighting, ventilation, dressing rooms/lockers, employee break areas, garbage/refuse storage, utility facilities, and insect/rodent control. Because not all states are aligned to the most current FDA Food Code (2009 with 2011 supplement), it is always best to first ensure facility designs meet the state requirements since states regulate food code and plan review design and issue food service permits to retail establishments.

For example, Georgia was one of several states that updated its food code to the most current FDA Food Code in the last 5 year and more recently updated its plan review requirements based on these rules called the Design, Installation and Construction Manual, Georgia Department of Public Health, Environmental Health, Food Service (Georgia 2012). This manual has 357 pages and provides detailed specifications for each of the areas described above including additional equipment specifications and templates that assist in the application process for new or renovation facilities construction. This manual is a good resource to learn more about how to design faculties based on FDA-aligned food code requirements and what regulatory expectations will be during operations (i.e., health department inspections often will be performed to verify these facility design specifications).

It is not the scope of this chapter to review each of these specifications for food safety facility design and how each contributes to prevention of food safety hazards. However, several of the more important hazards have been (and continue to be) identified in retail food service establishments according to the FDA in its report on the occurrence of foodborne illness risk factors in selected institutional food service, restaurant, and retail food store facility types (FDA 2009). Of the most common risk factors known to cause a foodborne illness in restaurants, cleaning and sanitizing food contact surfaces and utensils, protecting food from environmental contamination, separating raw animal foods from ready-to-eat foods (sometimes called flow of food), adequate hand washing facilities (and access), and improper holding of foods (temperature control) are each directly linked to facility design (and or maintenance of design) and should be emphasized here. The highest three risk factors for a foodborne illness found in retail establishments is improper holding/time and temperature, poor personal hygiene, and contaminated equipment/protection from contamination; only one is not directly related to facility design—poor personal hygiene.

In order to address these important food safety risk identified and quantified by the FDA, a retail food service facility space design should organize all equipment and space needs based on the flow of food (see Fig. 6.1 as example) that will maximize separation of raw animal foods from ready-to-eat foods and minimize cross contact flow of these two foods (i.e., improper raw food prep in areas of ready-to-eat food prep and improper movement of ready-to-eat foods toward raw food prep). Depending on the menu and requirements for extensive food preparation (washing, cutting, mixing, cooking) in each retail food establishment and the capacity of storage needs, it should be a priority to design complete separation of raw animal and ready-to-eat foods (e.g., different refrigerators for each and separate sides of the

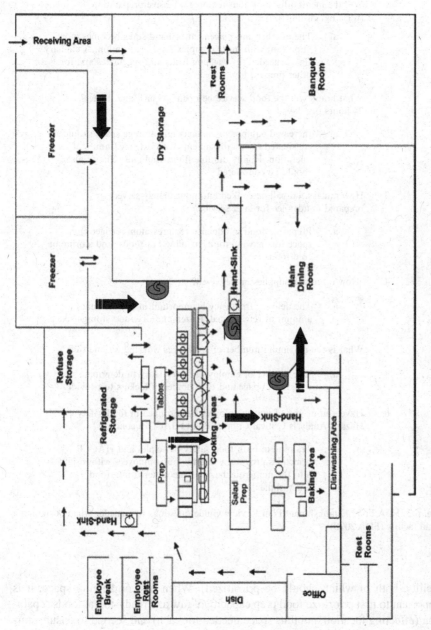

Fig. 6.1 Design of a retail facility to enable separation and safe flow of raw to RTE food movement/preparation

Questions to Consider:

1. Will the menu offer food that requires extensive preparation
    (washing, cutting, mixing, etc.)?

    a.   The number and placement of hand sinks becomes more
         important with more complex food preparation. A culinary
         sink is needed for washing fruits and vegetables and for
         other preparation.

2. What hours will the food service be open?... lunch and dinner?...
    24 hours per day?

    a.   Increased equipment capacity and storage space should be
         considered for establishments with extended hours of
         operation. Highly durable floor, wall and ceiling finishes
         should be considered.

3. How much food will be cooked and immediately served, or
    prepared in advance for later service?

    a.   Preparing food in advance requires more refrigeration
         space for thawing foods, cooling hot foods, and storing of
         cold foods.

4. How often will supplies be delivered?

    a.   The delivery frequency is important in determining the
         amount of refrigerated, frozen and dry food storage space.

5. What is the maximum number of employees working on one shift?

    a.   The number of employees is necessary to determine
         work/aisle space and the number of lockers to provide.

6. Have you or any of your employees been trained in food safety or
    Hazard Analysis Critical Control Point (HACCP) concepts?

    a.   Training in both food safety principles and HACCP
         principles provides you and your employees with insight
         into the numerous hazards encountered in a food
         establishment.

Fig. 6.2 FDA Food Establishment Plan Review Guide questions to consider when designing a
retail facility (FDA 2000)

facility, both of which should be prioritized). When first organizing space, it is
important to first prioritize food prep capacity of raw and ready-to-eat foods separation (effecting location and thus space needed for each) and second to ensure storage capacity after (and close to) receiving area to ensure all raw ingredients can be
stored separate from dry goods and ready-to-eat foods (Fig. 6.1). The FDA Food
Establishment Plan Review Guide provides guidance in this area that can help

SECTION II

REGULATORY AUTHORITY COMPLIANCE REVIEW LIST AND APPROVAL/
DISAPPROVAL FORM

REGULATORY AUTHORITY COMPLIANCE REVIEW LIST

	SAT.	UNSAT.	N/A	INSUFF. INFORM.
1. Food Preparation Review				
Raw food prep table(s) (as menu dictates)	( )	( )	( )	( )
Raw food prep sink(s) (as menu indicates)	( )	( )	( )	( )
Adequate refrigeration	( )	( )	( )	( )
Adequate hot holding facilities	( )	( )	( )	( )
Adequate hot food preparation equip.	( )	( )	( )	( )
Vacuum packaging (HACCP plan)	( )	( )	( )	( )
2. Utensil & Equipment Storage				
Clean	( )	( )	( )	( )
Soiled	( )	( )	( )	( )
Counter mounted equip.	( )	( )	( )	( )
Floor mounted equip.	( )	( )	( )	( )
Vacuum packaging equip.	( )	( )	( )	( )
Bulk Food	( )	( )	( )	( )
Self service	( )	( )	( )	( )
Salad	( )	( )	( )	( )
Hot/Cold Buffet	( )	( )	( )	( )
3. Kitchen Equipment				
Spacing between units or wall closed; moveable, or adequate space for easy cleaning	( )	( )	( )	( )

Fig. 6.3 FDA Food Establishment Plan Review Guide often used by state regulatory authorities to determine facility design requirement approval (FDA 2000)

facility engineers with questions they should consider for space design necessary to meet this food safety need (e.g., Fig. 6.2) and a helpful checklist (Fig. 6.3) designed for regulatory authorities but useful here, which more specifically defines design requirements necessary to meet food code requirements.

Another important risk factor FDA identified that is related to facilities design is adequate hand washing facilities (and access to them). Hand washing faculties should be integrated into the flow of food design. Because hand washing is the most critical means to reduce pathogens on hands (and thus cross contamination of ready-to-eat foods), each hand washing station should form a barrier (i.e., employees can easily wash hands between food prep task in two areas) between raw animal foods and ready-to-eat foods (see gray hand sinks Fig. 6.1). Because another hazard is associated with team member health and personal hygiene (e.g., employee who has undiagnosed norovirus infection), it is also important to ensure a hand

Work space & aisles sufficient	( )	( )	( )	( )
Storage 6" off floor	( )	( )	( )	( )
Countertops & cutting boards of suitable material	( )	( )	( )	( )
Self serve food area adequately protected	( )	( )	( )	( )
Approved thermometer for each refrigerator & freezer, and for taking food temperatures	( )	( )	( )	( )

4. Finish Schedule

Kitchen	( )	( )	( )	( )
Bar	( )	( )	( )	( )
Food Storage	( )	( )	( )	( )
Other Storage	( )	( )	( )	( )
Toilet Rooms	( )	( )	( )	( )
Dressing Rooms	( )	( )	( )	( )
Garbage & Refuse Storage	( )	( )	( )	( )
Mop Service Area	( )	( )	( )	( )
Ware washing Area	( )	( )	( )	( )
Walk-in refrigerator & freezers	( )	( )	( )	( )

5. Plumbing

Cross Connections	( )	( )	( )	( )
Water Supply	( )	( )	( )	( )
Sewage Disposal	( )	( )	( )	( )
Hand Sinks	( )	( )	( )	( )
Dishwashing & Pot Sinks	( )	( )	( )	( )
Grease Traps	( )	( )	( )	( )
Service/Janitorial Sinks	( )	( )	( )	( )
Hot Water	( )	( )	( )	( )

6. Physical Facilities

Dressing Rooms	( )	( )	( )	( )
Separate Toxic Storage	( )	( )	( )	( )

Fig. 6.3 (continued)

washing sink is located between the restroom facilities and the food prep facilities (at entry into the kitchen from dining area/restrooms). Location of hand washing sinks away from food preparation areas (including ice and beverage handling/prep) is also an important design consideration in the flow of food design to ensure hand washing activities do not cross contaminate food. If a hand washing facility must be located near any food prep, a stainless steel barrier (with height defined by risk of splash from hand washing, generally 12 in.) should be installed.

Laundry Facilities	()	()	()	()
Linen Storage	()	()	()	()
Lighting	()	()	()	()
Food Storage	()	()	()	()
Dry Storage Goods	()	()	()	()

7. Refuse & Pest Control

Garbage & Refuse Storage	()	()	()	()
Insect & Rodent	()	()	()	()
Control Measures	()	()	()	()

8. Ventilation

Exhaust Hoods	()	()	()	()
Ventilation	()	()	()	()

9. Employee Restrooms

Location	()	()	()	()
Number _____	()	()	()	()
Soap Dispensers	()	()	()	()
Hand Drying	()	()	()	()
Lavatories	()	()	()	()
Water Closets	()	()	()	()
Urinals	()	()	()	()
Hot & Cold Water Provided	()	()	()	()
Waste Receptacles	()	()	()	()

10. Patron Restrooms

Location	()	()	()	()
Number _____	()	()	()	()
Soap Dispensers	()	()	()	()
Hand Drying	()	()	()	()
Lavatories	()	()	()	()
Water Closets	()	()	()	()
Urinals	()	()	()	()
Hot & Cold Water Provided	()	()	()	()
Waste Receptacles	()	()	()	()

Fig. 6.3 (continued)

Two other important risk factors identified by the FDA's (2009) study were inadequate protection of food from environmental contamination and improper holding of foods. These two risk factors could easily be associated with employee behaviors (e.g., not covering foods during storage and/or storing raw animal foods over ready-to-eat foods, which would together increase risk of food contamination). However, improper facilities design could also contribute to inadequate protection of food from environmental contamination due to placement of, for example, produce prep sinks (where produce is rinsed and cut) next to dishwashing three compartment sinks (where dirty dishware is sprayed off before washing). Likewise, inadequate improper holding of foods could be caused simply by lack of refrigeration or freezer capacity leading to storage of foods on floors due to storage capacity issues.

Supplier Food Manufacturing Facilities

It will most likely be difficult to specify food safety specific facilities design in a supplier manufacturing faculties, many of which likely already exist. Therefore, certification of supplier facilities should be performed using one of the food safety GFSI standard schemes (BRC Global Standard for Food Safety, CanadaGAP, FSSC 22000 Food Products, Global Aquaculture Alliance Seafood Processing Standard, Global G.A.P, Global Red Meat Standard, IFS, PrimusGFS, and SQF) that evaluate a facility design as part of the operation certification process to ensure a safe environment for food production. This can also give the food safety management team confidence that the facilities are designed for proper cleaning and sanitation and to meet all regulatory standards in the design of a manufacturing facility. However, the food safety management team may also be able to specify new production lines for its ingredients/products and/or designate prohibition of specified allergens or other ingredients (e.g., gluten) on its product lines or from the facility (e.g., top eight allergen-free facility).

· Other factors to consider when visiting a supplier facility to determine if it can easily produce safe food are related to the equipment and placement of equipment in and around the designated production lines. This includes clearly defined flow of food for separation of ingredients from finished products, allergen control, and cleaning and sanitation design especially for clean-in-place equipment (CIP) and storage of chemicals for cleaning (including secure storage and traceability of all chemicals and pesticides). One factor that is often overlooked is the quality of the air in the production area of the facility. Although it may be difficult to specify air quality for many ingredients/products (and not necessary), some foods like fresh-cut produce including apples/pears may have a high probability of yeast/mold contamination simply due to air quality which can easily be remedied with air filtration systems (designing clean air rooms). Simply controlling air quality can lead to decrease spoilage of many perishable foods possibly increasing shelf life.

Food Defense (Security) and Facilities

Food defense is defined as the efforts to *prevent human intentional contamination* of food products by biological, chemical, physical, or radiological agents that are not reasonably likely to occur in the food supply. It is not the intention of this chapter to cover all aspects of food defense nor regulatory requirements (although they are directly linked and will likely be required under the Food Safety Modernization Act), but it is important for the food safety management program to consider the security of a food manufacturing facility it buys its ingredients/products from as an additional means to prevent hazards (even lower probable ones). The best means for the food safety management team to be prepared for any likely food defense issues is to ensure its retail and supplier manufacturing facilities have integrated food defense security specifications (defined below) AND it has the proper systems to provide surveillance for product defects, investigations of possible contamination, and recall methods to remove ingredients/products from its retail units within 2 h or sooner (discussed in Chap. 4) if a food tampering situation is evident. The information below is only a guide to help initiate thinking on the kinds of preventive measures each facility type may take to minimize the risk that food under its control will be subject to tampering or other criminal or terrorist actions.

Retail Facilities

The FDA recommends in its guidelines (FDA 2007a, b) that a food retail business, specifically for all retail units, should review its current procedures and controls; study the potential for tampering or other criminal or terrorist actions within its facilities; and make appropriate changes to prevent them. The FDA guidelines are designed to focus retail businesses on each part of the supply chain under their direct control (e.g., distribution and deliveries) to minimize the risk of tampering or other malicious, criminal, or terrorist action at each part. FDA-recommended guideline include a focus on *management* (preparing for the possibility of tampering or other malicious, criminal, or terrorist actions; investigation of suspicious activity; and initiating an evaluation program); *human element—staff* (screening (prehiring, at hiring, post-hiring), daily work assignments, identification, restricted access, personal items, training in food security procedures, unusual behavior, staff health)); *human element—public* (e.g., contractors, supplier representatives, delivery drivers, customers, couriers, pest control representatives, third-party auditors, regulators, reporters, kitchen tours); *facility* (physical security, storage and use of poisonous and toxic chemicals (e.g., cleaning and sanitizing agents, pesticides)); and *operations* (incoming products, storage, food service and retail display, security of water and utilities, mail packages, access to computer systems). The FDA guidance also contains a food defense self-assessment tool that is a helpful start in measuring the capability of a retail unit food defense capabilities (FDA 2007a, b), and Fig. 6.4 shows the facility-related physical security and storage checklist that can be used to measure the capabilities of a retail food facility to minimize the risk that food under its control will be subject to tampering or other criminal or terrorist actions.

Facility

Physical security

- ☐Y ☐N ☐N/A ☐Don't know – Protect non-public perimeter access with fencing or other deterrent, when appropriate

- ☐Y ☐N ☐N/A ☐Don't know – Secure all doors, windows, roof openings/hatches, vent openings, ventilation systems, utility rooms, ice manufacturing and storage rooms, loft areas and trailer bodies, and bulk storage tanks for liquids, solids and compressed gases to the extent possible

- ☐Y ☐N ☐N/A ☐Don't know – Use metal or metal-clad exterior doors to the extent possible when the facility is not in operation, except where visibility from public thoroughfares is an intended deterrent

- ☐Y ☐N ☐N/A ☐Don't know – Minimize the number of entrances to non-public areas

- ☐Y ☐N ☐N/A ☐Don't know – Account for all keys to establishment

- ☐Y ☐N ☐N/A ☐Don't know – Monitor the security of the premises using appropriate methods

- ☐Y ☐N ☐N/A ☐Don't know – Minimize, to the extent practical, places in public areas that an intruder could remain unseen after work hours

- ☐Y ☐N ☐N/A ☐Don't know – Minimize, to the extent practical, places in non-public areas that can be used to temporarily hide intentional contaminants

Fig. 6.4 Excerpt from V. Appendix: Food Defense Self-Assessment Tool for Retail Food Stores and Food Service Establishments in *Guidance for Industry: Retail Food Stores and Food Service Establishments: Food Security Preventive Measures Guidance*. *Note:* This is only a partial checklist taken from this guidance document; FDA recommends users to become familiar with the guidance document before using this tool

Supplier Facilities

First, all suppliers you do business with should already be registered according to the requirements of the Registration of Food Facilities Under the Public Health Security and Bioterrorism Preparedness and Response Act of 2002 (70 FR 57505). This regulation requires all facilities that manufacture/process, pack, or hold food,

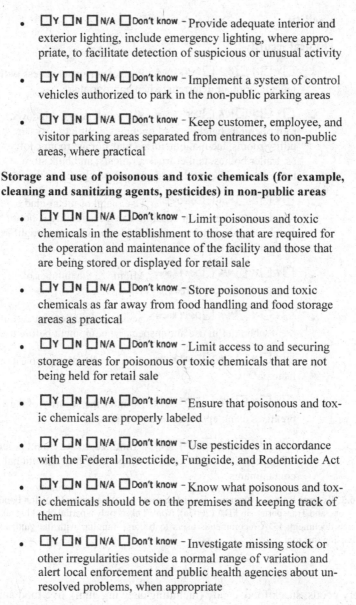

- ☐Y ☐N ☐N/A ☐Don't know – Provide adequate interior and exterior lighting, include emergency lighting, where appropriate, to facilitate detection of suspicious or unusual activity

- ☐Y ☐N ☐N/A ☐Don't know – Implement a system of control vehicles authorized to park in the non-public parking areas

- ☐Y ☐N ☐N/A ☐Don't know – Keep customer, employee, and visitor parking areas separated from entrances to non-public areas, where practical

Storage and use of poisonous and toxic chemicals (for example, cleaning and sanitizing agents, pesticides) in non-public areas

- ☐Y ☐N ☐N/A ☐Don't know – Limit poisonous and toxic chemicals in the establishment to those that are required for the operation and maintenance of the facility and those that are being stored or displayed for retail sale

- ☐Y ☐N ☐N/A ☐Don't know – Store poisonous and toxic chemicals as far away from food handling and food storage areas as practical

- ☐Y ☐N ☐N/A ☐Don't know – Limit access to and securing storage areas for poisonous or toxic chemicals that are not being held for retail sale

- ☐Y ☐N ☐N/A ☐Don't know – Ensure that poisonous and toxic chemicals are properly labeled

- ☐Y ☐N ☐N/A ☐Don't know – Use pesticides in accordance with the Federal Insecticide, Fungicide, and Rodenticide Act

- ☐Y ☐N ☐N/A ☐Don't know – Know what poisonous and toxic chemicals should be on the premises and keeping track of them

- ☐Y ☐N ☐N/A ☐Don't know – Investigate missing stock or other irregularities outside a normal range of variation and alert local enforcement and public health agencies about unresolved problems, when appropriate

Fig. 6.4 (continued)

as defined in the law, for consumption in the United States, to be registered with the FDA. Examples of "food" in this law include dietary supplements and dietary ingredients, infant formula, beverages (including alcoholic beverages and bottled water), fruits and vegetables, fish and seafood, dairy products and shell eggs, raw agricultural commodities for use as food or components of food, canned and frozen foods,

Facility

Physical security

- ☐Y ☐N ☐N/A ☐Don't know – Protect perimeter access with fencing or other deterrent, when appropriate

- ☐Y ☐N ☐N/A ☐Don't know – Secure all doors, windows, roof openings/hatches, vent openings, ventilation systems, utility rooms, ice manufacturing and storage rooms, loft areas, trailer bodies, tanker trucks, railcars, and bulk storage tanks for liquids, solids, and compressed gases, to the extent

- ☐Y ☐N ☐N/A ☐Don't know – Use metal or metal-clad exterior doors to the extent possible when the facility is not in operation, except where visibility from public thoroughfares is an intended deterrent

- ☐Y ☐N ☐N/A ☐Don't know – Minimize the number of entrances to restricted areas

- ☐Y ☐N ☐N/A ☐Don't know – Secure bulk unloading equipment when not in use and inspect the equipment before use

- ☐Y ☐N ☐N/A ☐Don't know – Account for all keys to establishment

- ☐Y ☐N ☐N/A ☐Don't know – Monitor the security of the premises using appropriate methods

- ☐Y ☐N ☐N/A ☐Don't know – Minimize, to the extent practical, places that can be used to temporarily hide intentional contaminants

Fig. 6.5 Excerpt from V. Appendix: Food Defense Self-Assessment Tool for Food Producers, Processors, and Transporters in FDA (2007a). *Note:* This is only a partial checklist taken from this guidance document; FDA recommends users to become familiar with the guidance document before using this tool

bakery goods, snack food, candy (including chewing gum), live food animals, animal feeds, and pet food. The food safety management program can use FDA guidance tools to evaluate a food manufacturer's commitment to food defense. Figure 6.5 shows the facility-related physical security and storage checklist that can be used to measure the capabilities of a supplier manufacturing facility to minimize the risk that food under its control will be subject to tampering or other criminal or terrorist actions.

Each of the FDA guidance documents are not considered regulatory requirements at this time, but many will likely be integrated into the new regulatory requirements in the Food Safety Modernization Act due to the wording within this legislation

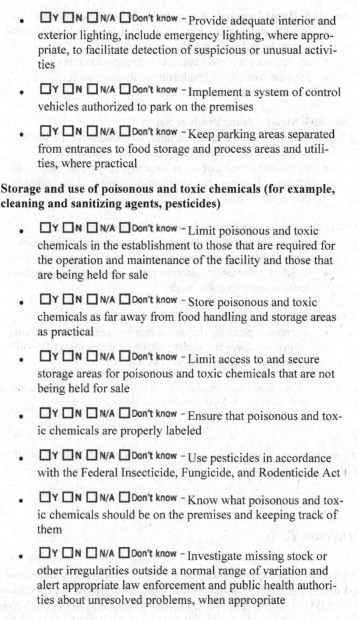

- ☐Y ☐N ☐N/A ☐Don't know – Provide adequate interior and exterior lighting, include emergency lighting, where appropriate, to facilitate detection of suspicious or unusual activities

- ☐Y ☐N ☐N/A ☐Don't know – Implement a system of control vehicles authorized to park on the premises

- ☐Y ☐N ☐N/A ☐Don't know – Keep parking areas separated from entrances to food storage and process areas and utilities, where practical

Storage and use of poisonous and toxic chemicals (for example, cleaning and sanitizing agents, pesticides)

- ☐Y ☐N ☐N/A ☐Don't know – Limit poisonous and toxic chemicals in the establishment to those that are required for the operation and maintenance of the facility and those that are being held for sale

- ☐Y ☐N ☐N/A ☐Don't know – Store poisonous and toxic chemicals as far away from food handling and storage areas as practical

- ☐Y ☐N ☐N/A ☐Don't know – Limit access to and secure storage areas for poisonous and toxic chemicals that are not being held for sale

- ☐Y ☐N ☐N/A ☐Don't know – Ensure that poisonous and toxic chemicals are properly labeled

- ☐Y ☐N ☐N/A ☐Don't know – Use pesticides in accordance with the Federal Insecticide, Fungicide, and Rodenticide Act

- ☐Y ☐N ☐N/A ☐Don't know – Know what poisonous and toxic chemicals should be on the premises and keeping track of them

- ☐Y ☐N ☐N/A ☐Don't know – Investigate missing stock or other irregularities outside a normal range of variation and alert appropriate law enforcement and public health authorities about unresolved problems, when appropriate

Fig. 6.5 (continued)

(see Fig. 6.6). Therefore, all food manufacturers should begin the process of using the current guidance documents if they have not already done so to prepare for the likely regulatory requirements. The food safety management program should also be familiar with food defense needs in its supply chain and consider alignment of its food manufacture facility specifications (or integrate food defense into its finished

Sec. 103- Hazard analysis & risk-based preventive controls:
- Identify and evaluate hazards that *may be intentionally introduced, including by acts of terrorism*
- Implement preventive controls to prevent hazards
- Monitor controls and maintain monitoring records
- Conduct verification activities

Sec. 105- Standards for Produce Safety
- Establish science-based, minimum standards for the safe production and harvesting of fruits and vegetables
- Consider hazards that occur naturally, may be unintentionally introduced, *or may be intentionally introduced, including by acts of terrorism.*

Sec. 106- Protection against *Intentional Adulteration*
- Issue regulations and guidance to protect against *the intentional adulteration of food*
- Conduct *vulnerability assessments of the food supply* and determine mitigation strategies

Sec. 108- National Agriculture & *Food Defense Strategy*
- A strategic planning document that will contain *food defense related guidance* for industry that is in the process of development, as directed, with USDA and DHS

Fig. 6.6 Example of language that contains expected rules related to *food defense* requirements for food manufacturers. Food Safety Modernization Act, (FDA 2012a, b, c)

product specification) as part of its responsibility to buy from suppliers that meet or exceed regulatory requirements.

Food Defense Tools

The FDA has all of the current food defense tools and resources for both retail facilities and food manufacturing/transportation facilities at http://www.fda.gove/fooddefense, and a CD-ROM is also available (*Food Defense Tools and Resources: It's Everybody's Business*) with all of the content as well (including retail-level employee training on food defense related to facilities issues, see FDA 2012a). The FDA provides a tool for updates on food defense related to future regulatory requirements at http://www.fda.gov/Food/FoodSafety/FSMA/default.htm. There are also several companies (e.g., Deloitte and Touche, LLP, ADM corporate security) expert in the area of food defense/security that have developed advanced consulting and development tools to support a food facility integration of food defense into its facility design.

More recently, the Food Safety Summit hosted a food defense workshop to help provide an overview of food defense for food manufacturers called "Food Safety Summit: Interactive Food Defense Workshop," and you can view the workshop on the FDA's FoodSHIELD Web site (FDA 2012a, b, c). The objectives of this workshop were to:

- Conduct a high-level overview of the various food defense tools and resources that have been developed by government
- Provide known industry leaders in the food defense arena an opportunity to share their stories on how these food defense tools and resources have been incorporated into existing operations
- Provide an "update" of the current status of the various food defense elements of the Food Safety Modernization Act

The presenters at this workshop were many of the experts in the field of food defense in addition to FDA experts and included a food manufacturer perspective in the application of food defense in facilities. This resource is a good starter into the subject matter, and the food retail business should initiate food defense in all its retail units and encourage food defense with its suppliers as a means to support government agencies in their work to protect the public health.

References

FDA (2000) Food establishment plan review guide. Available via internet at http://www.fda.gov/Food/FoodSafety/RetailFoodProtection/ComplianceEnforcement/ucm101639.htm

FDA (2007a) Guidance for industry: retail food stores and food service establishments: food security preventive measures guidance. Available via internet at http://www.fda.gov/Food/GuidanceComplianceRegulatoryInformation/GuidanceDocuments/FoodDefenseandEmergencyResponse/ucm082751.htm

FDA (2007b) Guidance for industry: food producers, processors, and transporters: food security preventive measures guidance. Available via internet at http://www.fda.gov/Food/GuidanceComplianceRegulatoryInformation/GuidanceDocuments/FoodDefenseandEmergencyResponse/ucm083075.htm

FDA (2009) FDA Report on the occurrence of foodborne illness risk factors in selected institutional foodservice, restaurant, and retail food store facility types (2009). Available via internet at http://www.fda.gov/Food/FoodSafety/RetailFoodProtection/FoodborneIllnessandRiskFactorReduction/RetailFoodRiskFactorStudies/ucm224321.htm

FDA (2012a) Food Safety Summit Workshop: Interactive Food Defense Workshop. Available via internet at http://www.fda.gov/Food/FoodDefense/EducationOutreach/ucm296729.htm

FDA (2012b) Employees FIRST: Food Defense Awareness for front-line food industry workers. Available via internet at http://www.fda.gov/Food/FoodDefense/ToolsResources/ucm295997.htm

FDA (2012c) Food safety modernization act. Available via internet at http://www.fda.gov/Food/FoodSafety/FSMA/default.htm

Georgia (2012) Design, installation and construction manual, georgia department of public health, environmental health, food service. Available via internet at http://health.state.ga.us/programs/envservices/FSPlanReviewManual.asp

Chapter 7
Execution and Verification

The expected responsibility of the food safety management program is to ensure all manufacture control systems which include all systems/specifications (including food safety SOPs), training and education, and facilities design are feasible and can be executed (i.e., validated that they can be performed as designed). A second but equal expectation is to verify that each manufacture control system (e.g., HACCP) is being continuously executed as designed, corrective actions are being made at the time of verification (enabling hazard prevention maintenance), and information collected is being used to continuously improve the hazard prevention. The food safety management team responsibilities should be to measure each manufacture control system under their area (e.g., supplier certification, retail unit third-party audit management, and restaurant third-party audits), to confirm that all systems are working together to prevent foodborne illnesses. Execution and verification should be measured by both self-assessment and third-party evaluation and the data then used to continuously monitor the effectiveness of the hazard prevention. The surveillance systems defined in Chap. 4 should validate this (i.e., no increase in reported ingredient/product defects).

Execution

Testing should be performed or other evidence gathered to validate each manufacture control system (including any food safety SOP) actually works to prevent the hazard before it is integrated (rolled out) into retail units and manufacturing faculties. This should include validation on the equipment, in the facilities, and performed by personnel trained at the level that will be performing the procedures and using the tools within the control system. Testing should be based on a statistical model (e.g., the right number of restaurants or manufacture production runs in the facility) and in the retail and manufacturing environments to ensure the manufacture control system is operationally feasible. This process is not new and is often followed by menu development teams when introducing a new product to retail units that include new procedures and equipment use.

H. King, *Food Safety Management: Implementing a Food Safety Program in a Food Retail Business*, Food Microbiology and Food Safety, DOI 10.1007/978-1-4614-6205-7_7, © Springer Science+Business Media New York 2013

A manufacture control system may appear to work well within a controlled kitchen or controlled test manufacturing environment with trained personnel performing the task. However, when put into the retail/manufacturing environment (where proper training/comprehension may be low or additional duties may be high), the control system may not be found to be operationally feasible in this environment. More important, when you attempt to verify this system later, you likely will find it as not being used properly to prevent the hazard (wasting time and money on both). For example, suppose you want to initiate a new manufacture control system to change surface sanitizer and require that all sanitizer solutions must be changed every 4 h due to the short shelf life of the sanitizer (e.g., chlorine-based sanitizers). You fail to validate if this procedure is operationally feasible in the retail environment, but assume that employees in all the retail units are performing this task (and therefore the hazard of cross contamination is being reduced). When you attempt to verify this control system by third-party audit of the retail units (by checking the sanitizer strength and when it was changed as an indicator that sanitizer is being maintained properly), you find that the majority of the retail unit sanitizer measurements are too low. Now, if you had validated this in several retail units first, you may have discovered that it was not feasible to change sanitizer solutions in all bottles, pails, etc. every 4 h due to time constraints and lack of proper tools, and this finding may have lead you to proposing a different sanitizer (e.g., quaternary ammonia-based sanitizer that only required change at end of the day) to achieve the same hazard reduction but now is operationally feasible (i.e., it can be executed properly to prevent the hazard).

In order to maximize the probability that a manufacture control system can be validated through testing in a retail or supplier environment, it must, of course, be tested in a controlled environment. When this has occurred and the system is defined as safe, it is then useful to test it in the retail or supplier environment but under the control (presence of a food safety management team member or designate) and with approval of the local health department (i.e., to comply with a change in menu or equipment regulatory compliance) in retail environments. This enables any changes to be carefully monitored and quickly identifies what training materials/tools work best to ensure consistency of the system by the employees of the retail unit. Once the control system and training methods have been validated in one unit, it is then recommended to validate it in enough retail units (statistical model should reflect a sample population of units that will perform the control system) after a defined period of time that will enable validation that the control system can be executed throughout all units as planned. This execution validation should be performed by a third-party audit of the control system and only after confirmation that all employees responsible for the system have been properly trained. This then sets the pattern for how the control system will be verified in the future when multiple units are using the control system as discussed below.

It is much easier to validate the execution of manufacture control systems in a retail environment (e.g., once you know the procedure is safe to test in units serving customers) than in a supplier manufacturing facility. Manufacturing facilities don't often produce multiple test runs of ingredients/products in multiple facilities. However, execution of a finished product specification (as a food safety manufacture control system) can be validated in a manufacturing facility by requesting the presence of the respective food safety management team member during the first production run of a retail business's specified ingredient/product production. This is necessary to also enable the business to test the ingredient/product against other specifications like nutritionals or sensory (taste) by the product development team and can be performed at the same time. The food safety management team member or designate can observe each required system of the finished product specification (e.g., allergen control) and pull sample ingredients/products off the run for further chemical or microbiological testing to ensure the control systems are working. The statistical sampling should be based on the population to represent batch-to-batch variability in a finished ingredient/product. Once this first production run is found satisfactory for the manufacture control system, the manufacturing facility can be asked to hold (not release) all ingredients/products from the first few days of a production run to cover most variables (e.g., employee shift changes, day parts, and cleaning and sanitation rotations). Once these ingredients/products meet the defined final product specifications expected to enable retail sale, like undeclared allergen testing, they may be released into the supply chain by the food safety management team. Any verification requirement should be defined based on these data. Like retail unit validation of execution, this process then enables proper verification to be performed as described below.

Verification

The validation of execution for all manufacture control systems in retail units and supplier manufacturing facilities will provide the detailed elements that must be verified (including how often they should be verified). The next duty of the food safety management team is to verify that all food safety requirements are being executed and sustained.

Supply Chain

Traditionally, a food retail business (as buyer) will verify that a manufacturing facility is following its manufacture control systems via a food safety management team member (or QA staff) visit of the facilities. This is normally done during a production run of its ingredients/products. Then the team will use third-party food safety audits (normally provided by the manufacturing facility) to verify FDA or USDA compliance to GMPs and GAPs. Both methods of verification are very valuable to ensure specific details set by the food safety management program are in place (e.g., undeclared allergen control) but can be expensive to the retail food business (travel support and personnel needed to cover the large number of manufacturing and distribution facilities in its supply chain) and the manufacturer (numerous third-party audits and multiple expectations from different buyers). Additional issues using only these methods include the frequency and audit credibility (i.e., is the third-party audit unbiased and data current) and who is credible to audit the facilities. More importantly, what happens when issues are identified to ensure corrective actions have been made and documented at the time of a third-party audit (with knowledge that any audit data is already days if not months old)?

A relatively new method that many retail food businesses are using to verify food safety manufacture control systems is called the Global Food Safety Initiative (GFSI). Third-party certification is not new, but until GFSI was created, there was no international food safety standard that most food retail businesses could require in all domestic and nondomestic manufacturing facilities in its supply chain. As discussed in Chap. 4, this method enables the buyer to select pre-certified manufacturing facilities that meet rigorous food safety standards. An analogy to this (if applied as a requirement for supplying a food retail business) would be if the FDA or USDA were able to visit each of your food manufacturing facilities you buy from every year, score the facility based on risk (like a local health department scores a retail facility), and require that the facility meet all its GMP requirements in order to be certified. Although there are several schemes within the GFSI, you should study which is the most appropriate scheme to the food manufacturing facilities you buy from. The current GFSI schemes are the BRC Global Standard for Food Safety, CanadaGAP, FSSC 22000 Food Products, Global Aquaculture Alliance Seafood Processing Standard, Global G.A.P, Global Red Meat Standard, IFS, PrimusGFS, and Safe Quality Food (SQF). Because each GFSI scheme is based on different manufacturing processes (e.g., raw meats, packaged foods) and some have more focus on different food commodities (e.g., produce vs. dairy production), a buyer can have more confidence in the scientifically sound (and industry-wide-recognized) risk-based verification of the most appropriate food safety manufacturing control systems.

All GFSI certification schemes ensure the more important food safety manufacture control systems (e.g., prerequisite systems described in Chap. 4) are in place at the time of the certification audit and establish an annual manufacture control systems verification process, based on the recertification audit for each certified facility (Fig. 7.1). For example, an SQF recertification audit frequency (Fig. 7.2) is based on three ratings (E = excellent, G = good, and C = comply) and two types of nonconformance (major and minor) after the initial certification audit (assuming the facility receives a certification via a C, G, or E). A third type of nonconformance rating is measured called a critical nonconformance (deemed a breakdown in a control at a critical control point, prerequisite program, or other process step judged likely to cause a significant public health risk that would likely lead to a class 1 or class 2 recall if corrective action is not taken or falsification of records relating to food safety controls is detected). If any critical nonconformance item is detected at the time of a certification or recertification audit, the certification body (SQF) will suspend or withdraw the facilities certification. If a facility has a certification suspended or withdrawn, there is an even higher audit frequency after recertification is achieved to ensure the facility is meeting all the food safety manufacture control system requirements.

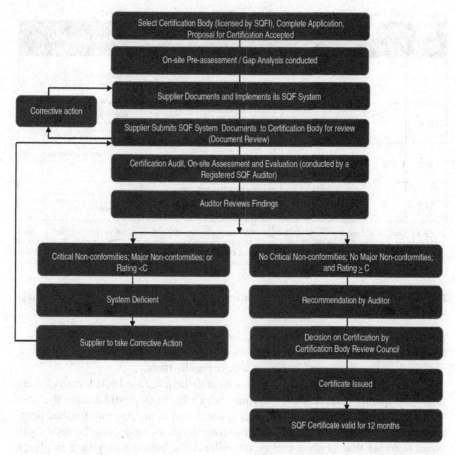

Fig. 7.1 Steps to achieve third-party food safety certification the GFSI scheme SQF (SQF 2000 Code, 2008)

Verification of more specific manufacturing control systems/specifications of the facility can be performed using corporate specific addendums to the GFSI certification schemes. Each addendum can be built into the annual recertification audit process specific to any additional systems/specifications in each facility the buyer requires (e.g., finished product spec that may include hold and release testing, allergen testing of product, or evidence of dated retained samples of its ingredients/products). Using GFSI schemes with addendums as a means to verify a food retail business's manufacture control systems/specification requirements allows the food safety management program to augment its verification resources (personnel and travel budget) toward higher risk manufacturing facilities (e.g., manufacturers that produce cooked protein products or a manufacturer that is identified via the number and degree of hazards and/or the number of ingredient/product defects that have occurred over time). It is important to note here that these addendums are not scored nor calculated as part of the certification audit grade. However, they can provide important additional information

Table 4 Determining the Audit Frequency (Audit Rating: **E** = Excellent; **G** = Good; **C** = Comply)

Audit Rating	Type of Non Conformance			Action	Audit Frequency
	Critical	Major	Minor		
C	-	-	-	Supplier to Correct all Non-conformances identified. Certification Body to verify Non-conformances are Corrected before Issuing the SQF 2000 Certificate of Registration.	6 months Surveillance until an appropriate Audit result is achieved
E/G	0	0	≤20	Supplier to Correct Non-conformance. Certification Body to verify Non-conformances are Corrected before Issuing the SQF 2000 Certificate of Registration.	12 months; otherwise 6 months surveillance until an appropriate Audit result is achieved
E/G	0	≤1	≤10	Supplier to Correct Non-conformance. Certification Body to verify Non-conformances are Corrected before Issuing the SQF 2000 Certificate of Registration.	12 months; otherwise 6 months surveillance until an appropriate Audit result is achieved
E/G	0	≤2	≤0	Supplier to Correct Non-conformance. Certification Body to verify Non-conformances are Corrected before Issuing the SQF 2000 Certificate of Registration.	12 months; otherwise 6 months surveillance until an appropriate Audit result is achieved

10.19.3.2 Once Certified the Audit frequency shall be amended depending on the type/number of Non-conformances detected at a Re-certification Audit and the overall rating achieved. The Suppliers Certificate of Registration shall be maintained provided the required conditions are met and the number of Non-conformances does not exceed the threshold level requiring the suspension (see 10.18.3) or withdrawal (see 10.18.4) of the Certificate of Registration.

Fig. 7.2 SQF auditing frequency based on type of prior nonconformance and audit ratings (SQF 2000 Code, 2008)

on annual risk for each manufacturing facility that can be used to trigger additional staff visits and/or third-party audits on a more regular basis.

GFSI certification audits can also significantly help the food safety management team (and quality team as well) determine which facilities should receive the most verification focus. This in turn will likely reduce cost of unnecessary finished product testing or visits to all food manufacturing facilities supplying the food retail business (other than general quality surveillance the business may have in place). Using GFSI schemes may also reduce cost of managing ingredient/product withdrawals or recalls. GFSI third-party certification would be expected to reduce some recalls and product withdrawals especially for undeclared allergens related to failure of allergen control systems.

Suppose you buy packaged chocolate milk from three different manufacturers that are each GFSI certified (rating of excellent) per requirements discussed above, but one also makes almond milk in the same facility. You have an addendum to audit the facility to verify your additional allergen specification (which includes requirements that the manufacturer not make almond milk in the same production room as your chocolate milk line) and perform test of all finished product for almond protein before release of your product to distribution. This manufacturer may be classified as a higher risk manufacturing facility, if, for example, the recertification audit notes several minor nonconformances in the area of allergen control and this facility received a G with three identical minor nonconformances the year before.

Because of the increased risk of a customer consuming chocolate milk with undeclared almond allergen, you may score this manufacturing facility as a higher risk supplier (but not the other two chocolate milk manufacturers) and perform additional verifications (and put this supplier on notice of such) at this facility. You may pull samples from distribution centers (before they are shipped to retail units) of the chocolate milk representative of several production runs from the facility and test them for almond protein as a precaution. You likely will have one of the food safety management team members visit this facility to verify all prerequisite allergen control systems/specifications are in place and verify the proper retained samples are present for each batch/lot production run.

Managing Supplier Food Safety Risk Through Verifications Data

Additional verification data from the food safety management programs' surveillance systems (described in more detail in Chap. 4; see Fig. 4.8) can be used along with all other verification data to measure the number and type of issues for all ingredient/product suppliers (through their manufacturers and distributors facilities data). These measurements can then be used to determine which facilities and/or distribution centers should get the most focus of the food safety management team due to risk of a food safety hazard failure. For example, suppose the chocolate milk suppliers facility (the supplier discussed in the product withdrawal scenario in Chap. 4) had, over the last 2 months, three retail units report product defects of spoiled milk taste, one SQF audit with CIP issues noted as nonconformance (but corrected), and one FDA warning letter (posted 30–60 days after an FDA audit in some cases). In addition to this, your quality sampling data (pulling product from distribution centers) showed several examples of spoiled product due to temperature abuse postproduction. Together, these verifications data would have induced the food safety management team to investigate the manufacturing facilities of this chocolate milk supplier and likely put product on hold well before a crisis arises at the retail level of the supply chain. If verification data shows the facility continues to produce defects in the product it makes even after intervention, the team would likely move production to a secondary supplier.

Of course the means to capture and analyze multiple inputs of data on each suppliers manufacturing facility is critical to the success of using verification data appropriately. A data capture system technology with reporting capabilities could help manage the measurements of each manufacturing facility (e.g., dashboards with reporting outputs like green, for approved for distribution; yellow, on alert with additional product testing required and/or visit by the food safety management team; and red, not approved for distribution/secondary supplier needed). Figure 7.3 shows an example of how the food safety management program might track risk in manufacturing facilities based on information received from verification of food safety control systems.

Several technology companies offer services to track recertification (or other food safety third-party) audits including some of the certification bodies (e.g., SQF). Others are able to tailor computer systems software to a business's specific manufacture control systems criteria. This could include tracking verification of

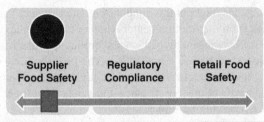

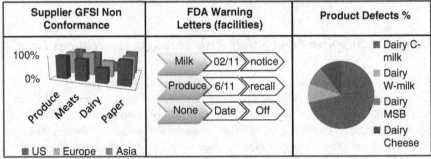

Fig. 7.3 Example concept for a computer software dashboard to display verification data in the supply chain and rate different supplier facilities based on food safety risk

finished product specifications from a facility via laboratory testing data capture (via electronic laboratory management system (LMS)) and other facilities' related data via a dashboard display. Some technologies can even provide automatic notice (via e-mail or voice mail) to alert the food safety management team, for example, when a manufacturer does not pass a GFSI scheme recertification audit or reports a specific number or type of nonconformances during a recertification audit. Thus, a verification monitoring system could be helpful to the food safety management team to focus its resources on risk and could be supportive of quality verification resource needs for the business as well.

Retail Units

All retail units should have both a regular self-assessment and third-party evaluation program as part of its food safety manufacture control systems verification. The food safety management program should develop retail self-assessment criteria based on its HACCP plans (e.g., CCPs during food prep measured daily) and the most current FDA Food Code inspection form with detailed "how to" instructions and correction actions (Fig. 7.4); performed at least monthly. It is critical that all corrective actions are defined, made, and documented during all self-assessments. These retail unit self-assessments then serve as a method to ensure each retail unit is checking food safety hazards and making corrections to ensure prevention methods are being used

FORM 3-A

Food Establishment Inspection Report

Page ____ of ____

As Governed by State Code Section XXX.XXX		No. of Risk Factor/Intervention Violations		Date ____
Do Good County		No. of Repeat Risk Factor/Intervention Violations		Time In ____
12344 Any Street, Our Town, State 11111		Score *(optional)*		Time Out ____
Establishment	Address	City/State	Zip Code	Telephone
License/Permit #	Permit Holder	Purpose of Inspection	Est. Type	Risk Category

FOODBORNE ILLNESS RISK FACTORS AND PUBLIC HEALTH INTERVENTIONS

Circle designated compliance status (IN, OUT, N/O, N/A) for each numbered item   Mark "X" in appropriate box for COS and/or R

IN=in compliance   OUT=not in compliance   N/O=not observed   N/A=not applicable   COS=corrected on-site during inspection   R=repeat violation

Compliance Status		COS	R	Compliance Status		COS	R
Supervision				**Potentially Hazardous Food Time/Temperature**			
1 IN OUT	Person in charge present, demonstrates knowledge, and performs duties			16 IN OUT N/A N/O	Proper cooking time & temperatures		
Employee Health				17 IN OUT N/A N/O	Proper reheating procedures for hot holding		
2 IN OUT	Management, food employee and conditional employee; knowledge, responsibilities and reporting			18 IN OUT N/A N/O	Proper cooling time & temperatures		
				19 IN OUT N/A N/O	Proper hot holding temperatures		
3 IN OUT	Proper use of restriction and exclusion			20 IN OUT N/A	Proper cold holding temperatures		
Good Hygienic Practices				21 IN OUT N/A N/O	Proper date marking & disposition		
4 IN OUT N/O	Proper eating, tasting, drinking, or tobacco use			22 IN OUT N/A N/O	Time as a public health control: procedures & record		
5 IN OUT N/O	No discharge from eyes, nose, and mouth			**Consumer Advisory**			
Preventing Contamination by Hands				23 IN OUT N/A	Consumer advisory provided for raw or undercooked foods		
6 IN OUT N/O	Hands clean & properly washed			**Highly Susceptible Populations**			
7 IN OUT N/A N/O	No bare hand contact with RTE food or a pre-approved alternative procedure properly allowed			24 IN OUT N/A	Pasteurized foods used; prohibited foods not offered		
8 IN OUT	Adequate handwashing sinks properly supplied and accessible			**Chemical**			
Approved Source				25 IN OUT N/A	Food additives: approved & properly used		
9 IN OUT	Food obtained from approved source			26 IN OUT	Toxic substances properly identified, stored, & used		
10 IN OUT N/A N/O	Food received at proper temperature			**Conformance with Approved Procedures**			
11 IN OUT	Food in good condition, safe, & unadulterated			27 IN OUT N/A	Compliance with variance, specialized process, & HACCP plan		
12 IN OUT N/A N/O	Required records available: shellstock tags, parasite destruction						
Protection from Contamination							
13 IN OUT N/A	Food separated & protected			Risk factors are improper practices or procedures identified as the most prevalent contributing factors of foodborne illness or injury. Public Health Interventions are control measures to prevent foodborne illness or injury.			
14 IN OUT N/A	Food-contact surfaces: cleaned & sanitized						
15 IN OUT	Proper disposition of returned, previously served, reconditioned, & unsafe food						

GOOD RETAIL PRACTICES

Good Retail Practices are preventative measures to control the addition of pathogens, chemicals, and physical objects into foods.

Mark "X" in box if numbered item is **not** in compliance   Mark "X" in appropriate box for COS and/or R   COS=corrected on-site during inspection   R=repeat violation

		COS	R			COS	R
Safe Food and Water				**Proper Use of Utensils**			
28	Pasteurized eggs used where required			41	In-use utensils: properly stored		
29	Water & ice from approved source			42	Utensils, equipment & linens: properly stored, dried, & handled		
30	Variance obtained for specialized processing methods			43	Single-use/single-service articles: properly stored & used		
Food Temperature Control				44	Gloves used properly		
31	Proper cooling methods used; adequate equipment for temperature control			**Utensils, Equipment and Vending**			
32	Plant food properly cooked for hot holding			45	Food & non-food contact surfaces cleanable, properly designed, constructed, & used		
33	Approved thawing methods used			46	Warewashing facilities: installed, maintained, & used; test strips		
34	Thermometers provided & accurate			47	Non-food contact surfaces clean		
Food Identification				**Physical Facilities**			
35	Food properly labeled; original container			48	Hot & cold water available; adequate pressure		
Prevention of Food Contamination				49	Plumbing installed; proper backflow devices		
36	Insects, rodents, & animals not present			50	Sewage & waste water properly disposed		
37	Contamination prevented during food preparation, storage & display			51	Toilet facilities: properly constructed, supplied, & cleaned		
38	Personal cleanliness			52	Garbage & refuse properly disposed; facilities maintained		
39	Wiping cloths: properly used & stored			53	Physical facilities installed, maintained, & clean		
40	Washing fruits & vegetables			54	Adequate ventilation & lighting; designated areas used		

Person In Charge (Signature)		Date:	
Inspector (Signature)		Follow-up: YES NO (Circle one) Follow-up Date:	

Fig. 7.4 FDA Model Food Code-based inspection form to use as a model for retail unit food safety verification audits (FDA 2012)

properly, and each unit will be in compliance to the most current food safety inspection criteria (of which most states have or will soon adopt as the criteria for food safety requirements for retail food establishments).

Some retail food businesses require reporting of food safety self-assessments to the food safety management program, while others allow the retail units to perform these audits but track the retail units' current health inspection grade/score. I would recommend a self-assessment program where the retail units are required to perform self-assessments but not report daily and monthly assessment data to the food safety management team (unless of course they need support). This model is based on selection of competent owners who demonstrate the responsibility of food safety in their units.

The third-party food safety evaluation of each retail unit should also be based on the most current FDA Food Code inspection form (FDA 2012) and performed at a minimum once a year (more often if needed based on performance against each criteria rather than score/grade). It may not be feasible to audit all CCPs within the time frame and cost of performing third-party audits in retail units, but some CCPs could be added as part of the audit (e.g., cooking CCPs). It is important that each third-party audit includes a process to ensure corrective actions for all foodborne illness risk factors (see Fig. 7.4) to ensure a food safety hazard is corrected. These corrective actions should be documented. The food safety management team should manage the reports (in collaboration with operations field staff) to verify that each retail unit is in compliance to all food safety requirements of the food safety management program. If both the self-assessment and third-party audits are based on the same criteria as recommended above (i.e., HACCP and FDA Food Code), then the food safety management team can correlate the data from both in analysis/work for continuous improvement of all food safety manufacture systems at the retail level of its business.

The food safety management team should analyze collective retail data for each food safety criteria representing all retail units in the organization. This will provide data to focus and prioritize current resources on those criteria that are not performing as required. For example, if the quarterly data shows that 90% of all retail units are failing a CCP for cooking a frozen meat that must be thawed before cooking (assuming of course each is making corrective actions and recooking the meat), the food safety management team would investigate the general cause of this failure (e.g., supplier is manufacturing the meat too large for the thawing platform).

A final important verification the food safety management team can perform is to visit the retail units and work a day or two performing the required food prep task and cleaning and sanitation SOPs within the facility. This is one of the best methods I found to discover risk not reported via other verification methods or to determine the root cause of food safety hazards reported through verification. When I wanted to learn more about reported dishwashing struggles in a retail unit, I would work a day washing dishes to see if I could follow the required SOPs and be in compliance to food code rules. This type of verification can also provide the data you need (personal experience) at a much lower cost than other methods necessary to influence and gain resources for improvement of food safety within the food retail business (discussed in more details in Chap. 9).

It is not the scope of this chapter to discuss all the line items to verify in each manufacture control system/specification in all supplier and retail facilities. Several of these systems may be verified as part of quality and finished product evaluations. It is my intent here to provide the most cost-effective means to verify both critical food safety hazards prevention and regulatory compliance in the supply chain and retail sides of the business with an added means to provide focus on the problem areas by each of the respective dedicated team members (the supplier food safety manager, the regulatory compliance manger, and the retail food safety manager) of the food safety management team described in Chap. 3. All of the food safety manufacture control systems described in Chap. 4 (see Table 4.1, Chap. 4) should be verified via HACCP and GFSI certification audits for suppliers and HACCP and FDA Food Code requirement audits for retail units.

References

FDA (2012) FDA Food Code 2009: Annex 7—model forms, guides and other aids. Available via internet at http://www.fda.gov/Food/FoodSafety/RetailFoodProtection/FoodCode/FoodCode2009/ucm188327.htm#form3a

SQF 2000 Code (2008) A HACCP-based supplier assurance

Chapter 8
Gap Analysis

The food retail business and its food safety management program should periodically be benchmarked against the most current regulatory requirements and industry food safety standards to determine if gaps exist in the program. Gap analysis of the food safety management program differs from the day-to-day verification of systems/specifications, training/education, and facilities design effectiveness. Gap analysis measures the food safety management program (with a focus on systems/specifications) within the food retail business against the most current benchmarked standards of food safety. Before a Gap analysis can be performed appropriately, the food safety management team must be established, and all components discussed in Chaps. 4 to 7 should be functional. It is assumed that all components of commitment (defined in Chaps. 2 and 3) to food safety have been addressed before a Gap analysis is initiated.

The Gap analysis should be performed by a third party to ensure an unbiased benchmark and include review of the management of food safety and all food safety documentation, systems/specifications, training/education, and facilities design areas of the food retail business based on a set of defined strategic objectives for each. The food safety management team should coordinate and review all deficiencies with an action plan prioritized on the level of risk identified. Gap analysis should be performed on a periodic basis (based on size and growth of the business) most effectively after the food safety management program is well established and used as the road map for program improvement. Ultimately, Gap analysis (as a program matures) should confirm that the food safety management program is functioning properly to prevent food safety hazards within a food retail business.

What Is a Gap Analysis and Why Is It Important?

A Gap analysis allows a food retail business to compare its current food safety management program and components (called strategic objectives here) against accredited food safety management standards and identify deficiencies or gaps. These gaps

H. King, *Food Safety Management: Implementing a Food Safety Program in a Food Retail Business*, Food Microbiology and Food Safety, DOI 10.1007/978-1-4614-6205-7_8, © Springer Science+Business Media New York 2013

could be failure in the current systems/specifications, training, facilities design, or methods of verification, for example, but could also identify new gaps that have developed over time based on the size and growth of the business. Once gaps have been identified, an action plan can be made to strategically improve management of food safety risk and business performance. A periodic Gap analysis can also significantly align the food safety management program to the business needs by identifying more cost-effective means to reduce hazards across all components of the business. A Gap analysis should be conducted by a third-party consultant or business with expertise in food safety management systems (e.g., a GFSI certification body or auditing firm/consultant) so the review is unbiased and provides a transparent assessment of the food retail businesses' food safety risk. The third party should be under legal obligation for confidentiality (contract), and the food retail business must already be committed (will provide resources even if out of annual budget cycle) to take action on the identified deficiencies before a Gap analysis is performed. A food retail business should not perform a Gap analysis if it is not committed to providing the resources (see Chap. 9) to enable action on identified gaps.

How to Design the Gap Analysis

Determine the Standard for All Strategic Objectives

The Gap analysis should review the systems/specifications, training and education, facilities design, and execution/verification for the retail, supplier, and regulatory food safety components of the food safety management program (see Chap. 1, Fig. 1.2). There is currently no single food safety management program standard that can be used to measure a food retail business program against. This book is a first attempt at defining this. Because the work of the food safety management program is centered around corporate management of food safety risk in the supplier, retail, and regulatory components of the program, I recommend three standards that can be used to develop strategic objectives necessary to perform the steps in a Gap analysis of the food safety management program (Fig. 8.1). First, the food safety clauses of GFSI can be used to define basic strategic objectives of a food safety management program (Fig. 8.2). The GFSI clauses have well-defined strategic objectives for what a food safety management program should manage. Although the strategic objectives of GFSI clauses are specific to the manufacture of food, they can be easily adapted/revised as an outline for the food retail business program's strategic objectives for corporate control systems here. For example, measuring the food safety program management against the standards for management policy, management responsibility, management systems, and document control could help identify deficiencies in these areas that may help the team better manage corporate control systems under its responsibilities.

Second, a GFSI-based scheme (use one of the GFSI schemes most appropriate for the majority type of food suppliers used) can be used to define the strategic objectives of the supplier food safety area of the business. Each of the GFSI schemes

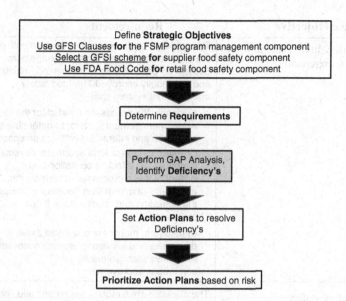

Fig. 8.1 Steps to perform a food safety Gap analysis of a food safety management program (FSMP) in a retail food business

define the general food safety management system requirements necessary for a food manufacturer (your suppliers) involved in the production, processing, transport, storage, and distribution of raw materials, ingredients, food products, and processed or prepared foods and beverages. It is best to choose only one that best fits your supplier food safety program. For example, if your supply chain is common to and buys many similar food commodities, you could choose one of the GFSI schemes (e.g., SQF, BRC, GRMS (Global Red Meat Standard)) based on the majority of supplier ingredients/products produced for your business.

Third, the most current FDA Food Code can be used as the strategic objectives for all retail food safety Gap analysis planning. Because you likely have already based all food safety systems and specifications, training and education, facilities design, and execution/verification on these rules, it will be healthy to perform a Gap analysis of the retail units' documented components in order to ensure these strategic objectives are being met. Carefully review all sections of the most current FDA Food Code with emphasis on the facility design (e.g., plan review), systems (e.g., HACCP), and training and education (e.g., employee personal hygiene) required to prevent food safety hazards in all retail units including catering and any mobile food service.

The food safety management team member responsible for the three areas of the program (regulatory compliance supplier food safety, and retail food safety managers) should provide detailed documentation of all manufacture and corporate control system standards (e.g., see Chap. 4, Table 4.1) of the business already established in the food safety management program. It is not the scope of this chapter to review all the possible standards you may use to set the strategic objectives and requirements for supplier food safety, retail food safety regulatory compliance, and food safety program

Strategic Objective	Requirements
Food safety management general requirements	The standard shall require that the elements of the organization's Food Safety Management System be documented, implemented, maintained and continually improved. The food safety management system shall: a) identify the processes needed for the food safety management system, b) determine the sequence and interaction of these processes, c) determine the criteria and methods required to ensure the effective operation and control of these processes, d) ensure the availability of information necessary to support the operation and monitoring of these processes, e) measure, monitor and analyze these processes and implement actions necessary to achieve planned results and continuous improvement.
Food safety policy	The standard shall require the organization has a clear, concise and documented food safety policy statement and objectives specifying the extent of the organization's commitment to meet the safety needs of its products.
Food safety manual	The standard shall require the organization has a Food Safety Manual or documented system having a scope appropriate to the range of business activities to be covered, including documented procedures or specific reference to them and describing the interaction of the related process steps.
Management responsibilities	The standard shall require that the supplier establish a clear organizational structure, which unambiguously defines and documents the job functions, responsibilities and reporting relationships of at least those staff whose activities affect food safety.

Fig. 8.2 Example strategic objectives developed to measure the food safety management program via Gap analysis using GFSI clauses (GFSI Guidance Document 2012)

management. These standards should be specific to each different food retail business and its respective risk (e.g., raw meats supplied to retail units vs. cooked, package ready-to-eat meats supplied to retail units) and must be carefully determined to fit each business need. It is highly recommended that you seek comparison of your food safety management program to other similar food retail business standards via

Management commitment	The standard shall require that the organization's senior management provide evidence of their commitment to establish, implement, maintain and improve the food safety system.
Management review	The standard shall require that the organization's senior management review the verification of the food safety system, HACCP Plan or HACCP based plans, at planned intervals, to ensure their continuing suitability, adequacy and effectiveness. The HACCP Plan shall also be reviewed in the event of any change that impacts food safety. Such a review shall evaluate the need for changes to the food safety system, including the food safety policy and food safety objectives.
Resource management	The standard shall require that the organization's senior management determine and provide, in a timely manner, all the resources needed to implment, maintain and improve the food safety system.
General Documentation	The standard shall require that documentation procedures are in place to demonstrate compliance with the standard and ensure that all records required to demonstrate the effective operation and control of its processes and its management of food safety are securely stored for a time period required to meet customer or legal requirements, effectively controlled and readily accessible when needed.
Specified requirements	The standard shall require that the organization ensure that, for all inputs to the process, items and services (including utilities, transport and maintenance) that are purchased or provided and have an effect on product safety, documented specifications are prepared, maintained, securely stored and readily accessible when needed. The standard shall require that a specification review process is in place.
Procedures	The standard shall require that the organization establish, implement and maintain detailed procedures and instructions for all processes and operations having an effect on food safety.
Internal audit	The standard shall require that the organization has an internal audit system in place to cover the scope of the food safety system, including the HACCP Plan or the HACCP based plan.

Fig. 8.2 (continued)

Corrective action	The standard shall require that the organization has procedures for the determination and implementation of corrective action in the event of any significant non conformity relating to food safety.
Control of non conformity	The standard shall require that the organization has effective processes in place to ensure that any product, which does not conform to food safety requirements, is clearly identified and controlled to prevent unintended use or delivery. These activities shall be defined in a documented procedure that is securely stored and readily accessible when needed.
Product release	The standard shall require that the organization prepare and implement appropriate product release procedures.
Purchasing	The standard shall require that the organization control purchasing processes to ensure that all externally sourced materials and services, which have an effect on food safety, conform to requirements. Where an organization chooses to outsource any process that may have an effect on food safety, the organization shall ensure control over such processes. Control of such outsourced processes shall be identified and documented within the food safety system.
Supplier performance	The standard shall require that the organization establish, implement and maintain procedures for the evaluation, approval and continued monitoring of suppliers, which have an effect on food safety.The results of evaluations, investigations and follow up actions shall be recorded.
Outsourcing	The standard shall require that,where an organization chooses to outsource any process that may affect food safety, the organization shall ensure control over such processes. Control of such outsourced processes shall be identified, documented and monitored within the food safety management system.

Fig. 8.2 (continued)

participation with industry-specific trade groups (e.g., National Restaurant Association, Food Marketing Institute, National Council of Chain Restaurants, and United Fresh Fruits and Vegetables). Many of these trade groups hold meetings and publish best practices to ensure food safety in a retail food business, and the professionals within the membership are a great resource to "pick up" standards for strategic objectives similar to their business and yours.

Complaint handling	The standard shall require that the organization establish, implement and maintain an effective system for the management of complaints and complaint data to control and correct shortcomings in food safety.
Serious incident management	The standard shall require that the organization establish, implement and maintain an effective incident management procedure, which is regularly tested for all products it supplies and covers planning for product withdrawal and product recall as required.
Control of measuring and monitoring devices	The standard shall require that the organization identify the measurement of parameters critical to ensure food safety, the measuring and monitoring devices required and methods to assure that the calibration of these measuring and monitoring devices is traceable to a recognized standard.
Food defense	The standard shall require that the organization has a documented risk assessment procedure in place to address food defense risks and establish, implement and maintain a system to reduce or eliminate the identified risks. The system shall cover GoodAgricultural Practices or Good Manufacturing Practices and shall be supported by the food safety system.
Product labeling	The standard shall require that the organization ensure that all product bears information to enable the safe handling, display, storage and preparation and use of the product within the food supply chain or by the consumer.

Fig. 8.2 (continued)

Measure Current Standing (Requirements) of Each Strategic Objective

Before the third-party agency performs a Gap analysis and, it should be provided the documental strategic objectives and respective requirements and demonstrate understanding of each, and both parties agree on its "fit" to the food safety Gap analysis. This should be performed using a Gap analysis planning table (Fig. 8.3 shows an example of an abbreviated table) that lists both the strategic objectives

Strategic Objective	Requirement	Deficiency	Action Plan
Systems: Product withdrawal and recall	All ingredients and products distributed to retail units must have date and time of manufacture and approved source identification	Approved fresh cut produce packaging found in retail units with no date and time of production identification	Supplier must immediately add label to all packaging with date and time of production- audit in 30 days to confirm
Training and education: corporate employees	All corporate field staff employees should be trained in the retail food safety management program requirements for retail units	Food safety training is assumed to be optional and 2/3's of the field staff have not received the most current retail food safety management requirements	Initiate retail food safety management requirements training for all field staff not trained within last two years
Facilities: Food defense: storage of hazardous chemicals and toxic substances in manufacturing facilities	All ingredient and product manufactures/distributors must have designated secure storage of all chemicals used for cleaning and sanitation/pest management	3 out of 10 distribution warehouses do not have secure storage, and residual pesticide containers were found in food storage areas	Distribution warehouses must immediately secure chemical storage- audit within 30 days to confirm 10/10 comply
Verification: Corrective and preventative action	All third party audits of retail units require immediate corrective action and documentation at the time of the audit (e.g., failed CCP).	Third party auditing firm was found documenting failed CCP's but not providing support to correct CCP at time of audit. No procedures for corrective actions were available to the auditing firm	Alert retail units on need to correct all CCP's at time of third party audit. Provide corrective action procedures of all retail CCP's to auditing firm, and require training of auditors- audit in 30 days to confirm

Fig. 8.3 Example elements from an abbreviated Gap analysis planning table for the supplier and retail components of the food safety management program. *Note*: It would be expected that a more comprehensive table would result from a complete Gap analysis of all manufacture control systems

and the food retail business's determined *requirements* of which all parties will work from during the Gap analysis. The third-party agency should then be asked to provide a proposal for how it will perform the Gap analysis and at what estimated cost and time. This should include a process to alert the food safety management team of any critical food safety issues it may identify that can be corrected immediately during any audits of supplier or retail facilities. Likewise, a food safety management team member should be designated as the lead business contact/ manager over the Gap analysis process to collect all data in real time (i.e., not waiting on a final report 3 months after staring a Gap analysis) to enable work on action plans that can be initiated with current resources within the food retail business. For example, if a supplier is identified that is not following your current requirements for labeling all products with date and time of production, the food safety management team can act on this deficiency immediately while others are still in review. Other deficiencies may not be quickly resolved and thus must be documented with action plans that include time line for resolution based on risk of the deficiency and resources available (see Chap. 9).

The third-party agency should have access to all food safety management program documentation for existing systems/specifications, training/education, facility design, and execution/verification components of the program for supplier food safety, regulatory compliance, and retail food safety components of the program. All documented retail food preperation procedures should also be made available to compare each against the requirements to ensure specific deficiencies can be identified and differentiated from training deficiencies. This is important because many of the deficiencies at the retail level may not be in the actual design in procedures, food safety SOPs, tools, or facility design, but could be due to a deficiency in how the employees are trained (e.g., training materials used and how training is verified).

The Gap analysis of the food safety management program should measure gaps within the three components (FSPM program management component, supplier food safety component, and retail food safety component—see Figs. 8.1) to cover all parts of food retail business functions (with one specific Gap analysis planning table for each). The Gap analysis is best performed with a recommended time line of 3 months. Phase one of the Gap analysis should be a third-party document review against all strategic objectives and requirements of the food safety management program (and how its managed using a planning table based on the GFSI clauses example in Fig. 8.2) with independent summary report provided to the food safety management team before phases two and three are initiated. This will ensure the third party is educated in the specific components of the businesses' food safety management program before they begin phase two and three below. It will also enable the food safety management team to identify any documents available but not routinely used/updated (e.g., crisis management procedures during flooding) so that the second and third phases of the Gap analysis will be comprehensive to the existing program.

Phase two should include document review and third-party audits of the supplier food safety and retail food safety components using the strategic objectives and requirements defined as the benchmark for food manufacturing at the supplier level (representative of all commodities the retail business purchases for its retail units) and retail unit operations using a GFSI scheme-based planning table for suppliers and FDA Food code-based planning table for retail units (see Fig. 8.3). It should not be necessary to audit all manufacturing facilities nor retail units in this process (this should be part of the program's routine verification component). However, it is important to gain insight through sampling each specific commodity, distribution process, and retail unit concept to ensure deficiencies can be discovered. An advantage of using an industry standard like GFSI for all suppliers and a third-party auditing agency certified to perform GFIS scheme audits for the planning table this phase of the Gap analysis is that it can be designed to target the higher risk commodities, higher rates of nonconformances, and those with the most significant expected deficiencies likely due to need for additional addendums specific to the food safety management program needs. Likewise, using the FDA Model Food Code inspection form (see Fig. 7.4, Chap. 7) as the means to measure all retail units will enable a comprehensive measurement of gaps in regulatory compliance as well.

Phase three of the Gap analysis (which will measure training/education and verification, i.e., perceptions vs. knowledge of food safety and food safety needs within the organization) should include interviews of all business managers over each business function (e.g., retail operations, purchasing, supply chain facilities design departments) including each team member of the food safety management program with previously designed questionnaires related to each strategic objectives and requirement within their business function (e.g., see Fig. 8.4). Additionally, a questionnaire for retail unit operators/managers should be formulated to address retail-specific strategic objectives and requirements. These questionnaires will serve two functions in the Gap analysis. First, it will provide insight on why a related deficiency exist in a specific strategic objective and assist you with developing a more specific action plan to ensure it will be sustained. For example, the operations department must support training requirements, may need to provide funding, and must provide accountability to its field staff to ensure compliance to food safety training requirements identified as a deficiency in the example action plan described in (Fig. 8.3; Training and Education). Second, the questionnaires will serve as additional education of the business leaders within the organization and lay the foundation for support of the work and likely resources to work on action plans.

Define the Deficiencies

It is important that the third-party agent performs all work on defining and reporting deficiencies according to the Gap analysis planning table. This should include all facility audits and interviews of staff within the food retail business.

This will ensure an unbiased/transparent assessment of requirements and deficiencies within all components of the food retail business. The deficiencies should be documented on the Gap analysis planning tables at each phase and provided to the food safety management team for review and development of the action plan. All data can be correlated during analysis of each Gap analysis planning table and reduce overlap of specific deficiencies within each.

Develop Action Plan to Resolve Each Deficiency

An action plan is a set of strategic steps that need to be taken for the food safety management team to resolve deficiencies identified by a Gap analysis. Each team manager responsible for program management of supplier food safety, regulatory compliance, and retail food safety should be responsible for developing the action plan for their respective area (e.g., Gap analysis planning table for suppliers is managed by the supplier food safety manager on the team). These managers can then

Strategic Objective	Question	Requirement	Deficiency
Systems/ Specifications: Food safety management	Is there a Food Safety manual?	A food safety manual should be maintained and include all manufacture control systems required in retail units including HACCP plans	50% of the retail operators were not aware of a food safety manual and thus not familiar of current food safety requirements
Training and education: employee food safety training	Is there a requirement for refresher training on food safety for all retail employees?	The program should designate when employees should be re-certified	None of the retail operators interviewed re-trained employees on updated food safety requirements
Facilities: design	Are the facilities designed to enable proper storage of employee personal belongings including medicines.	Facilities should be designed to include individual storage lockers for each employee to lock medicines and personal belongings away from food and access by other employees	Only new facilities contain lockers with locks. All older facilities only have coat closets
Verification:	Are you aware of any internal food safety assessments program for retail units?	All retail units should verify all HACCP and other food safety manufacture control systems via self assessment according to prescribed frequency	No internal food safety self assessment tool exist specific to the retail food safety requirements of the business. However, retail operators use regular refrigeration temperature monitoring.

Fig. 8.4 Example questions from an abbreviated GAP analysis planning questionnaire table to measure retail unit operator awareness and identify deficiencies at the retail level of the business. *Note*: It would be expected that a more comprehensive list of questions for both retail operators and department managers of the food retail business would be developed based on both industry and government standards

meet with each of their respective cross functional teams (see Fig. 3.3, Chap. 3) first to determine the most cost-effective means to jointly resolve each deficiency. It is likely that many resolutions will be made by simply reinforcing current requirements by additional means (e.g., communications, and field staff audits) allowing focus of current resources toward higher-risk deficiencies.

Going Forward

Each time you perform a Gap analysis (e.g., every 3–5 years) and all deficiencies are resolved (including program management), you should see continuous improvement in the management and prevention of food safety hazards within the business and have a clear picture (with data to support this) of what the resource needs are to sustain the investment made in food safety. Some deficiencies will require additional resources in people and funding to develop new systems/specification within the business. Many of these will require additional research and project management to develop and test the execution of new food safety systems/specifications. The Gap analysis should form the basis (road map) of the necessary data to influence the business and acquire the necessary resources in annual planning cycles until all deficiencies are resolved, prioritizing resolution based on risk.

Reference

GFSI Guidance Document (2012) Guidance document part III: scheme scope and key elements, sixth edition, issue 3, version 6.2. Available via internet at http://www.mygfsi.com/technical-resources/guidance-document/issue-3-version-62.html

Chapter 9
Influence and Resources

The food safety management program is a mandatory business function of a food retail business. Of all the business deliverables within an organization, the work performed by the food safety management team is most easily supported after a serious food safety issue occurs within the organization. Likewise, the program becomes less noticed and more difficult to support when there have been no direct customer-related food safety issues within the business even when the teams work is the likely cause of this outcome (through prevention of food safety issues). In order to influence and gain resources in a food retail business, the food safety management team should generate specific data on risk, prioritize the needs based on the highest risk, develop the methods, cost and plan to reduce the risk, and then work to influence the organization to support the risk reduction work through resources and people. Because other departments (e.g., marketing, purchasing, legal, and finance) have equally valid competitive needs for resources and people based on the mission of the business (funds for growth, facility improvements, marketing, development of new products, prevention of injury liability, etc.), the food safety management team should demonstrate the dollar value (e.g., reduced cost via prevention of withdrawals and recalls) of their work to the business beyond prevention of foodborne illnesses. The food safety management team can also show value via increasing profit (e.g., by preventing unnecessary food recalls and withdrawals that drive up cost) and leverage key relationships within and outside the business to enable resources to enhance its effectiveness to the business.

Influence

The work of the food safety professional working in the retail food business is similar in many ways to the work of a public health professional. Both must demonstrate need (influence) and seek funding (resources) to develop and implement effective interventions to prevent foodborne illnesses. A public health professional likely has significant influence, when risk data supports threats to public health, on their

H. King, *Food Safety Management: Implementing a Food Safety Program in a Food Retail* 103
Business, Food Microbiology and Food Safety, DOI 10.1007/978-1-4614-6205-7_9,
© Springer Science+Business Media New York 2013

department managers, directors, and the organization simply due to the mutual mission of the public health professional and the public health organization (e.g., to prevent illnesses in their state or nation, a.k.a., the CDC, USDA, or FDA). The influence of a food safety professional in a retail food business is oftentimes more difficult because the defined mission of the business is to sell more food and increase profits (sometimes perceived as sells minus cost of the food safety management program to the business).

The food safety management program structure defined in Chap. 3 should already be positioned to influence the business through its work on cross-functional teams and in supporting the business functions within the organization (Fig. 3.3, Chap. 3). This alignment is critical to the influence of the program on the business so that the focus is on mutual ownership of the food safety responsibilities and the collaborative effort to seek and fund cost effective solutions to deficiencies. Likewise, the organization must be committed to continuous improvement of food safety even when there have been no food safety issues by enabling the food safety management team to research food safety risk and make proposal for improvements as part of the normal planning processes within the business. It is not the scope of this chapter to discuss all the means to influence and acquire resources in a food retail business, but to describe common methods that have been successful via business relationships. It is recommended to the reader to benchmark these and other methods within industry trade group forums and through professional relationships with other food safety professionals in other food retail organizations.

Define and Prioritize the Specific Food Safety Deficiencies Within the Business

As discussed in Chap. 3, the primary duties of the food safety management team are the routine study of the hazards within the supplier and retail areas of the business, defining the deficiencies that lead to these hazards, develope systems/specifications, training/education, and facility design, and ensure it the execution and verification to prevent these hazards. In order for the team to influence the organization to spend new money on hazard prevention, the team should prioritize all hazards based on their highest probability (i.e., highest risk). Any newly identified hazard during regular third-party audits/field staff verification at manufacturer or retail units should be addressed immediately, and the food safety management program should already have resources (or be allowed to go out of budget with justification) to resolve. When the food safety management program has completed a Gap analysis and generated a planning table (see Fig. 8.3, Chap. 8 as example), this table should be used first in the development of solutions for each deficiency/action plan.

There are two main factors involved in a food safety management professionals influence on the business to make decisions to support food safety action plans (or any food safety recommendation that identifies a need to prevent a significant hazard). First, the credibility of the food safety professional is important and

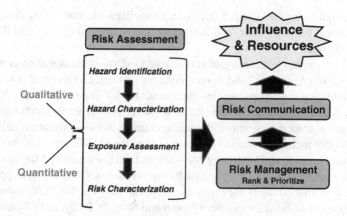

Fig. 9.1 Risk analysis used by the food safety management team to influence and gain resources to prevent food safety hazards

oftentimes respected by the business due to the transparency in communication and pursuit of resources that are only necessary to prevent significant hazards (in partnership with other business function stakeholders to reduce cost—see below). Second, the food safety management professional can provide data to support the need by ranking the hazards based on probability (hazard × probability = risk) which also provides transparency in the food safety management programs plans and enables the business to prepare for the plans.

Many organizations including government regulatory and investigative agencies tasked to prioritize foodborne illness prevention strategies use risk analysis as part of this process. According to experts in risk analysis design and application (Yoe 2012), risk analysis is defined as a process for making decisions under uncertainty. Risk analysis is made up of three task: risk assessment (describing the risk), risk management (doing something about the unacceptable risk), and risk communication (talking about the risk). Food safety management professionals can use risk analysis as a means to influence and gain resources by qualitatively or quantitatively describing a risk to the business, ranking the risk according to probability and consequences (i.e., in order to prioritize those risk and resource needs first), and communicating the priory risk/needs as part of the budget planning process to the business (Fig. 9.1).

It is not the scope of this chapter to describe how to perform risk analysis, specifically risk assessments, because the application of this task differs significantly depending on the risk being measured. For example, one may choose to perform a qualitative risk assessment using data from within the business (e.g., how many product withdrawals have been caused by yeast/mold spoilage) or quantitative risk assessment using published data on microbiological risk (e.g., risk of *Listeria monocytogenes* in processed milk) to make decisions in the organization. Likewise, many (but not all) of the deficiencies identified in a Gap analysis (or during routine verifications of food safety systems and specifications) may require additional risk assessment in order to develop the appropriate scope of the action plan necessary to correct the deficiency (see Chap. 8, Fig. 8.3). This will enable many of the deficiencies to be evaluated based on their food safety risk and enable prioritization of the items in the action plan.

Advanced training is recommended to enable food safety management professionals to perform risk analysis, and several colleges and universities offer risk analysis courses including one sponsored by Joint Institute for Food Safety and Nutrition (JIFSAN 2012). The JIFSAN Institute is a jointly administered, multidisciplinary research and education program (with training courses, including those online, on food safety risk) that includes research components from the FDA Centers for Food Safety and Applied Nutrition and Veterinary Medicine and the University of Maryland. Three additional references that complement each other and are useful tools in the application of risk analysis in food safety are *Primer on Risk Analysis* (Yoe 2012), *Microbiological Risk Assessment in Food Processing* (Brown and Stringer 2002), and *Microbial Risk Analysis of Foods* (Schaffner 2008). More detailed information and useful tools on risk communication (and perception of risk) as a means to influence stakeholders and support risk management are worthy of further study in these references.

Once the risks have been characterized clearly (for example based on each deficiency identified in a planning table, Chap. 8, Fig. 8.3 or through routine verifications data analysis), there are several methods to rank order and thus prioritize the risk so that action plans can be prioritized for obtaining resources. Many risks can be ranked simply based on published data showing the probability of the hazard is high, and these should be ranked first in the priority of action plans. Many other hazards can be resolved through risk communication strategies through cross-functional team participation with other business functions within the business (e.g., communicating the deficiency in food safety training in retail units to the training department can influence the department to gain resources and establish a training verification program).

Some risks are not so easily compared and require other means to rank them for priority based on more defined criteria. These risks can be ranked, based on several characteristics of the deficiencies and their possible solutions, by the food safety management team. One useful method, called the enhanced criteria-based ranking process, has been used by many organizations to rank risk based on defined criteria of the risk and then enable prioritization of action plans based on risk. This process was first developed by the Plant Epidemiology and Risk Analysis Laboratory of the Animal Plant Health Inspection Service, USDA (Yoe 2012) and is useful as a means to rank order food safety deficiencies based on how the business defines the risk.

First, a planning table is established to list the strategic objectives, requirements, and deficiencies that are not easily managed through current resources in the business. For example, there may be several hazards identified that will require significant cost to the business, and each needs to be ranked in order of probability (risk) and cost to enable the food safety management team to prioritize which to seek resources for first. These planning tables can be derived from the Gap analysis planning tables described in Chap. 8 and re-listed according to which will require more resources in order to resolve.

Strategic Objective	Requirement	Deficiency	Action Plan	Rank
Systems/ Specifications: Cleaning and sanitation	All dish ware must be cleaned, sanitized, and dried before use in food prep.	Dish ware in three compartment sink is not being consistently washed, rinse, and sanitized.	Replace three compartment sinks used to hand wash dishes with mechanical ware washing equipment	**HHH**
Cleaning and sanitation	All food contact surfaces must be cleaned and sanitized before food prep.	Surface sanitizer is not used properly due to requirement to mix before use	Require pre-moistened disposable wipes with sanitizer	**HHM**
Approved source	All produce must be from food safe sources	Produce is ordered from distributors who do not have identity of produce source	Develop managed produce distribution program	**HMH**
Training and education: Documentation	All procedures to manage food safety in the retail units should be documented and maintained to enable training and education of food safety managers	There is no food safety manual where program requirements are documented	Develop food safety web site to document/ maintain all food safety requirements	**LML**

Fig. 9.2 Example list of ranked proposed action plans from an abbreviated planning table and enhanced criteria-based ranking process used to prioritize risk and gain resources. Note: It would be expected that a more comprehensive table would be generated by the food safety management program specific to each component of the business (e.g., supplier or retail food safety manufacture control systems prioritization)

The process to rank each and answer which action plan should have the highest priority for resources has several defined steps (measured below as example and shown in Fig. 9.2):

1. A limited number of science-based criteria most often used to prioritize food safety risk are chosen to define each deficiency and its proposed action plan. These criteria should be limited to known risk (based on data) to more easily score each. For example, the food retail business may consider these three criteria to score each deficiency and action plan:

   (a) Foodborne illness outbreak occurrence
   (b) Regulatory compliance violations (low health scores/grades)
   (c) Lost sales volume in retail units

2. Each criteria (a–c) is given a high, medium, or low value according to its probability and consequences within the retail food business:

    H = high probability and high hazard
    M = lower probability but higher hazard
    L = lowest probability and no hazard

3. Each of the four (Fig. 9.2) deficiencies and their action plans are then scored for each of the three criteria in #1 above using data acquired by the food safety management team:

    *   Replace three compartment sinks used to hand wash dishes with mechanical ware washing equipment:

        –   1a = H, 1b = H, and 1c = H; Rank = **HHH**

    *   Require pre-moistened disposable wipes with sanitizer:

        –   1a = H, 1b = H, and 1c = M; Rank = **HHM**

    *   Develop managed produce distribution program:

        –   1a = H, 1b = M, and 1c = H; Rank = **HMH**

    *   Develop food safety web site to document/maintain all food safety requirements:

        –   1a = L, 1b = M, and 1c = L; Rank = **LML**

4. Each action plan is then prioritized in order it will be pursued (e.g., HHH = highest priority) for resources in the planning table (Fig. 9.2).

In this example, the food safety management team would pursue resources for replacement of all three compartment sinks used to hand wash dishes with mechanical ware washing equipment because its ranking among all action plans shows it has the highest risk to the organization based on the three criteria: (1) foodborne illness outbreak occurrence highly likely, (2) regulatory compliance violations (low health scores/grades) highly likely, and (3) lost sales volume in retail units highly likely. Of course, this is only a simple example of an enhanced criteria-based ranking process, and its value would directly correlate to the credibility of the data used to determine risk (e.g., retail data showed that when dishes were not cleaned and sanitized properly, there were 10^3 number of indicator bacteria (coliforms) on dishes used to prep fresh food). Enhanced criteria-based ranking is actually a type of qualitative risk assessment that can be effectively used to prioritize work needed on deficiencies and used to communicate risk as part of the risk management duties of the food safety management program.

Collaborate with Business Function Stakeholders to Define How to Implement Action Plans

One of the best means to influence change within a business is by collaborative agreement with other departments within the organization that the change is in the best interest of each respective department's mission. Most food safety action plans fall into this category, and the food safety management team can reduce cost and gain buy-in/collaboration with other departments to influence need for resources to make change (including people needs and fit on the right team). For example, suppose the organization's business analysis team in the finance department has been tasked to find areas within the business to reduce cost. During this time, the food safety management team has identified a deficiency in the cleaning and sanitation of dishware using three compartment sinks (e.g., dishware is not consistently being cleaned and sanitized properly) in all its retail units. This issue is likely to grow into a significant food safety risk if not changed soon (Fig. 9.2). The business analysis team discovers that significant cost is incurred when using three compartment sinks due to waste in water use and labor (including training), chemical, and electric use (control of hot water use) throughout the retail side of the business.

During collaborative research on the means to accomplish the food safety action plan, the cross-functional team discovers that a mechanical dish machine reduces significant cost (labor, water, chemical, electric) to the retail business (with return on investment in 6 months) and ensures all dishes are cleaned and sanitized significantly reducing this food safety risk in the business. During presentation of the action plan to the facilities department, the department discovers that installation of the new mechanical dish machine in all retail units will add back an additional 15 ft^2 (average) available food prep space to the kitchen.

When the food safety management team begins to seek resources for this change (capital equipment, installation, maintenance, training cost), the cross-functional need and thus the influence on the organization is significant in that the investment in the action plan will both reduce cost, enhance product production, and improve food safety. Of course, there will likely be support for the expected additional 15 ft^2 by several departments (e.g., product development department desires to add new equipment for new products) including the food safety management program needs (e.g., to improve separation of raw and ready-to-eat food prep if needed). Together, the business case for implementing this one food safety action plan is strong and likely to be supported by the food retail business.

It is important to prioritize all action plans based on risk and cost and then enable input by all respective business function managers on this prioritization before you begin to seek to influence within the organization. Transparency in this process is important to ensure trust and prevent the appearance of using other departments to gain influence. However, when there is no mutual need evident and the risk is high or growing, the responsibility of the food safety management team is to pursue the action plan.

Test to Validate Cost Benefit of the Action Plan to the Business

Food safety action plans that are not mutually beneficial to another department (or the benefits are not evident during research on solutions) and are prioritized as higher risk should be pursued through further research to define cost benefit to the organization. It is not recommended to speculate on cost nor accept vendor definitions on expected costs because you will be responsible (and must justify) for any differences after you influence the organization to make a change. Generally, this can be performed in a similar manner as in the retail unit or manufacturing systems testing to ensure execution described in Chap. 7.

The food safety management team should identify the tool/procedure to reduce the hazard, implement the change within the facilities (ensuring competency in training), and validate the change is being used properly and consistently in multiply units before measuring cost. Cost analysis should be performed on average unit expenditures (including labor if needed) by the business analysis department or other third-party financial expert and performed over a period of time that will represent the maximum use of the tool/procedure.

Oftentimes, research to define the true cost benefit of implementing an action plan will generate additional benefits not visible to the food safety management team during development. Let's go back again to the restaurant scenario in Chap. 2, where Sara the restaurant owner implemented a new disposable sanitizing wipe to replace cloth towel use (e.g., action plan in Fig. 9.2) due to the risk of storing cloth towels in water. Suppose this disposable sanitizing wipe was part of an action plan developed to address a deficiency in how all retail units improperly store cloth towels used to clean and sanitize food contact surfaces (e.g., spreading germs rather than removing them). Suppose during testing of the new disposable wipe in 30 retail units, it is discovered that, on average, the new wipe is more expensive to the retail unit when compared to maintaining cloth towels (laundry) and sanitizer chemicals in containers designated to store cloth towels. However, when the disposable wipes are used to clean and sanitize restaurant dining room tables, labor cost in preparing tables for change in customer (often referred to as turning tables in the restaurant business) is reduced, and customers perceive higher cleanliness of the dining room. When this additional benefit is calculated (sales and customer loyalty), the overall benefits now equal the increased cost, and the cost becomes neutral.

Translate Risk into Cost for the Organization Before Seeking Resources

In some cases, the cost of an action plan has no other benefit other than the more important reduction of the food safety hazard and prevention of a foodborne illness. It is then the responsibility of the food safety management team to communicate this risk and expected cost (carefully calculated based on actual use data) to initiate this action plan and seek the resources even without collaborative business function partners or positive cost:benefit results. Although the business leaders of the organization (if educated as discussed in Chap. 5) are likely to clearly understand the risk to the business (foodborne illness and/or outbreak), it is helpful to also show the cost of not implementing the action plan in business language (e.g., lost sales, increased cost of claims, and loss of brand equity). This will ensure that the food safety management team is not perceived by colleagues in the business as trumping all other business functions with unsubstantiated risk (e.g., people will die) and foster collaborative work on action plans, the majority of which will require the work and resources of other business functions within the business to succeed.

Resources

Traditional to most businesses, the food safety management team must compete with other business functions within the food retail business for available money and people in order to perform its duties through an annual planning process. The resources available are always limited and many times also restricted to a prior budget allowance for each business function. So equally important to "how to" obtain traditional resources (via influence discussed above) is managing resources well including sourcing nontraditional resources.

Managing Resources

A food safety management program requires a detailed budget process to ensure all current program needs are supported annually and additional resources are available to support new food safety action plans that arise from food safety verifications, research on risk, and Gap analysis. Each of the food safety management team members should have an individual budget to support required work in their business function area (business travel expenses, professional memberships, continuing education). Most of the cost within a food safety management program (after people and travel cost and assuming training/education and facilities design cost are within those respective business function departments) is centered around the cost of food safety corporate control systems and the execution/verification of food safety across all business functions. It is sometimes more difficult to acquire additional resources to implement new food safety action plans within the organization unless resources are managed well.

Nontraditional Resources

Many of the food safety companies (those that develop products to prevent food safety hazards and/or cleaning and sanitation chemicals/tools) work closely with retail food businesses to evaluate current and/or new products or services. These companies are often willing to provide resources in money and people to test their current products/services within a retail environment in order to validate the value of their product/service and help measure cost. Once the food safety management team has identified the probable solution to a deficiency and developed an action plan that requires a new tool/service, the team can source the best manufacturer for this tool/service and leverage this process in partnership with the training/education (to validate procedures) and purchasing business functions (negotiate cost) to generate the data necessary to support budget request to implement this action plan. If the data supports the action plan resolution and the cost is agreed upon, the food safety management team is already positioned to roll out the new action plan to all retail units. In many cases, the food safety company will provide resources for this communication and assist in the roll out of the tool/service as part of the business to business partnership.

Some food safety companies are interested in working with a retail food business (specifically in the retail unit environment) to test new products/services before they launch the products/services for sale to the industry. This provides the company with a more realistic environment to evaluate their product/service (after regulatory authorities have approved it in a state where the test will be performed) and enables the food safety management program to fund research on probable solutions to food safety action plans. Both parties can agree (under contract) that the data will be available for use by the food safety company (without endorsement) to aid in its internal and external product/service marketing (e.g., data showed 99% prevention of cross contamination) in return for the resources to fund the test that may result in a contract to purchase the product/service.

Let's suppose the retail food business franchisor of Sara's restaurant (going back to the scenario described in Chap. 2) desired to require all its 1,000 restaurant franchisees to use the new disposable wipes that Sara helped develop with a wipes manufacturer. However, the food safety management program did not have the resources to show the business the value of the new wipes, and it was challenged by the other departments that the issue was due to training and not operational feasibility of using cloth towels to clean and sanitize food contact surfaces. The food safety management team could partner with the wipes manufacturer to develop new procedures (SOP's for proper use) and test the product in its restaurants. In return for the resources to test the wipes (e.g., product and distribution cost, support, third-party evaluations, testing environmental surfaces, and surveys to determine value), the food safety management team offers the use of the third-party analyzed data for the food safety companies internal use (e.g., marketing the results). The food safety management team doesn't contract to roll out the wipes as a new requirement, but states it will use the data to seek support (and resources to do so) if the data supports value to the food retail business.

This type of collaboration for nontraditional resources can help the food safety management program evaluate new technologies, products, and services to resolve food safety deficiencies and provide the necessary data to show cost and benefits of the action plans to enable additional resources (via budget request) for the program. Many of these business to business relationships also benefit the retail unit owners/operators with more improved SOPs to reduce food safety hazards while also helping the food safety businesses that sell these items to gain the knowledge they need for improving the products and services for the food retail industry. I am convinced that more of these business to business relationships should be encouraged as a means to foster food safety product/services development within the food retail industry.

References

Brown M, Stringer M (2002) Microbiological risk assessment in food processing. CRC, Boca Raton

JIFSAN (2012) Available via internet at http://jifsan.umd.edu/

Schaffner DW (2008) Microbial risk analysis of foods. ASM, Washington, DC

Yoe C (2012) Primer on risk analysis. CRC, Boca Raton

Chapter 10
Partnerships with Public Health Officials

The food safety management program within a food retail business and the regulatory (FDA, USDA, state environmental health/health departments) and investigative agencies (CDC, state epidemiology investigations departments) have a common goal: to prevent retail customers from getting a foodborne illness. From the public health professionals' point of view, it is both their career mandate and their organization's mission to protect customers from foodborne illnesses; from the food safety management team professionals' point of view, in addition to customer safety, it builds loyalty, trust, and brand equity and can lead to increase in sales. Because of this common goal to prevent retail customers from getting a foodborne illness, improving partnerships between industry and government food safety professionals can significantly improve public health and the retail food businesses bottom line.

Partnerships begin with a food retail businesses focus on meeting and exceeding all regulatory requirements (in all retail units and through influencing food manufacturer compliance) with transparency to public health officials in how the organizations retail units and its manufacturers interpret and comply to regulatory requirements. Likewise, knowledge of how a foodborne disease outbreak is investigated is also key to enabling effective partnerships that can benefit a food retail business. This can enable more efficient foodborne illness investigations and protect the business from being unintentionally associated with a foodborne illness claims. Serving on regulatory/industry committees (e.g., food code rules committees) at the state and federal level and through the Conference for Food Protection (CFP) fosters partnerships between food safety professionals to find solutions that benefit both the public health and business. Developing working relationships with public health professionals at government- and industry-sponsored food safety forums (sharing knowledge and working together on understanding the cause of foodborne disease outbreaks) also enables joint efforts to develop new methods to reduce hazards (e.g., ability to comply to food code rules with operationally feasible SOPs) together.

H. King, *Food Safety Management: Implementing a Food Safety Program in a Food Retail Business*, Food Microbiology and Food Safety, DOI 10.1007/978-1-4614-6205-7_10, © Springer Science+Business Media New York 2013

Regulatory Compliance as Partnership

The most important action a food retail business can take to ensure strong partnerships with public health officials is to enable all retail units and require (as a buyer) all suppliers to meet or exceed current regulatory requirements. When a food retail business requires its retail units and suppliers to meet its manufacture control system requirements (and these meet or exceed regulatory requirements), this business has already partnered with public health by helping to ensure the safety of these products (and likely other products its manufacturers produce) as they enter commerce. Of course, some regulatory requirements will lag the most current science and knowledge on hazard prevention simply due to the steps and time required to validate each as a new regulatory rule (e.g., the FDA food code is updated on average every 5 years). Likewise, many states (as discussed below) have different food code rules, and sometimes different interpretations of how these rules should be followed. Therefore, it is important for the food safety management team to be versed in these rules and interpretations in any state where its retail units operate.

Understand and Support Foodborne Disease Investigations for the Benefit of Public Health

As discussed in Chap. 3, the burden of foodborne diseases in the United States continues to have significant impact on the food retail business through the efforts and cost it must spend to prevent known hazards. The CDC estimates that 1 in 6 Americans gets sick from a foodborne illness every year, and these illnesses are caused by both known foodborne pathogens and unspecified agents (CDC 2012). Unspecified agents causing foodborne illnesses are defined as those that cause acute gastroenteritis, but the agent and food have not yet been identified (e.g., microbes, chemicals, or other substances not known to be in food). In fact, there are an estimated larger percent of foodborne illnesses, hospitalizations, and deaths caused by unspecified agents (80%, 56%, and 56%, respectively—see Fig. 10.1) than there are for the known pathogens of foodborne diseases (CDC 2012). Many of these unspecified agents will likely be attributed to specific foods in the near future due to improving investigation methods and a focus on attributions by the CDC in its task to reduce the burden of foodborne illnesses in the United States.

Likewise, many of the outbreaks of foodborne diseases associated with retail sales of a contaminated food continue to cause illnesses and death many months after the contaminated food is identified, recalls are initiated, and the public is notified (see Fig. 1.1, Chap. 1). Foodborne illness outbreak investigations must therefore be an area where food safety professionals in retail food businesses and regulatory/investigative agencies improve partnerships to reduce number of cases of illness during the earliest phases of an outbreak investigation.

CDC Estimates of Foodborne Illness in the United States

FINDINGS

CDC 2011 Estimates

CDC estimates that each year roughly 1 in 6 Americans (or 48 million people) gets sick, 128,000 are hospitalized, and 3,000 die of foodborne diseases. The 2011 estimates provide the most accurate picture yet of which foodborne bacteria, viruses, microbes ("pathogens") are causing the most illnesses in the United States, as well as estimating the number of foodborne illnesses without a known cause.* The estimates show that there is still much work to be done—specifically in focusing efforts on the top known pathogens and identifying the causes of foodborne illness and death without a known cause.

Reducing foodborne illness by 10% would keep about 5 million Americans from getting sick each year.

CDC has estimates for two major groups of foodborne illnesses:

Known foodborne pathogens— 31 pathogens known to cause foodborne illness. Many of these pathogens are tracked by public health systems that track diseases and outbreaks.

***Unspecified agents—** Agents with insufficient data to estimate agent-specific burden; known agents not yet identified as causing foodborne illness; microbes, chemicals, or other substances known to be in food whose ability to cause illness is unproven; and agents not yet identified. Because you can't "track" what isn't yet identified, estimates for this group of agents started with the health effects or symptoms that they are most likely to cause—acute gastroenteritis.

To estimate the total number of foodborne illnesses, CDC estimated the number of illnesses caused by both known and unspecified agents. We also estimated the number of hospitalizations and deaths caused by these illnesses. Table 1 provides the estimates due to known pathogens, unspecified agents, and the total burden.

Table 1. Estimated annual number of domestically acquired foodborne illnesses, hospitalizations, and deaths due to 31 pathogens and unspecified agents transmitted through food, United States

Foodborne agents	Estimated annual number of **illnesses** (90% credible interval)	%	Estimated annual number of **hospitalizations** (90% credible interval)	%	Estimated annual number of **deaths** (90% credible interval)	%
31 known pathogens	9.4 million (6.6–12.7 million)	20	55,961 (39,534–75,741)	44	1,351 (712–2,268)	44
Unspecified agents	38.4 million (19.8–61.2 million)	00	71,878 (9,924–157,340)	56	1,686 (369–3,338)	56
Total	47.8 million (28.7–71.1 million)	100	127,839 (62,529–215,562)	100	3,037 (1,492–4,983)	100

National Center for Emerging & Zoonotic Infectious Diseases
Division of Foodborne, Waterborne, and Environmental Diseases

CS218786-A

Fig. 10.1 Differences between known and unspecified (unknown) causes of foodborne illnesses in the United States (CDC 2012)

There is a business case to be made also for improving partnerships and working together to improve systems to identify contaminated food during foodborne disease investigations. For example, in 2008, the FDA announced a national recall of red roma, red plum and red round tomatoes, and any other products containing these raw commodities (FDA 2008a). FDA lifted the warning one month later and went on to issue a new warning against raw jalapeno and raw serrano peppers from Mexico (FDA 2008b). Over 1,500 people became ill, 21% were hospitalized, and two died (Barton Behravesh et al. 2011) from contaminated produce during this outbreak. Although the tomato industry was reported to have suffered the most significant loss, food retail businesses suffered significant loss as well due to recall of all associated tomatoes and lost sales; the National Restaurant Association reported its members loss over $100 million (Meyerson 2009). Although food safety professionals in industry and regulatory/investigative agencies could argue one or the other is to blame for the cost of this outbreak, the facts are that if the industry had better means to identify source (via trace back) of produce sold at retail (see Product Traceability Corporate Control System, Chap. 4, Table 4.1) and the government agencies had more resources to rule out uncontaminated produce associated during case control analysis of the outbreak, significant cost could have been avoided. Both industry and regulatory/investigative food safety professionals would have to agree that better systems to trace tomatoes (and all other fresh produce) back to the farm and manufacturer, and track it from farms to food retail businesses is needed. Both the CDC and FDA would more than likely have identified the cause and source of the outbreak sooner if such a system exsisted, but more importantly, this would have enabled retail food businesses to continue to serve safe tomatoes (produce) with this knowledge (i.e., confidence their source of tomatoes was not part of the outbreak associated tomatoes, and they could demonstrate proof via trace back documentation).

Be Prepared to be a Part of a Foodborne Disease Investigation

Partnerships in foodborne illness investigations are first enabled by a foundation of well-defined and documented manufacture and corporate control systems (outlined in Chap. 4, Table 4.1). If and when an investigation leads to a retail facility (one of yours that sold the product to a customer), you will need to know and provide the documented procedures, systems (food safety SOP requirements) in place to receive, store, prepare, hold, and sell all foods. Public health officials will likely use a form similar to that shown in Fig. 10.2 (see Fig. 10.3 for completed form) to collect information on the flow of food prep in the facility (as a means to identify potential hazards) for any implicated food sold by the retail unit. By providing documented facility design, systems, and food prep procedures (including HACCP plans and verification methods) to public health officials during the investigation, it will reduce the time necessary to perform the investigation within your facility and improve the knowledge of the investigator about what they should see (behaviors of employees and methods used) within the facility.

FLOW PROCESS OF IMPLICATED FOOD -Form G			Complaint No.	
Name of Establishment	Person in Charge at Time of Analysis		Title	
Address			Date and time of Analysis	
Product(s) Evaluated (Include brand, code, date received)	Physical Appearance		pH	a_w

Diagram flow process of operation (Insert temperatures and time of processes or delays and make appropriate symbol at exact point in operation.)

Symbols to use in diagram:

+ Likelihood of growth	O Survival likely	⚠ Inital contamination likely.	⚠ Contamination by equipment/ utensils
− No growth	× Likelihood of destruction	▽ Worker/person contaminated	
∨ Vegetative cell	s - Bacterial spore		

Investigator		Title	Date

Fig. 10.2 Form likely used by local public health officials to investigate a foodborne illness claim and/or outbreak in a retail food service establishment. Reprinted with permission from Procedures to Investigate Foodborne Illness (Sixth Edition—2011) (Copyright held by the International Association for Food Protection, Des Moines, Iowa, USA. Available for purchase at http://www. foodprotection.org)

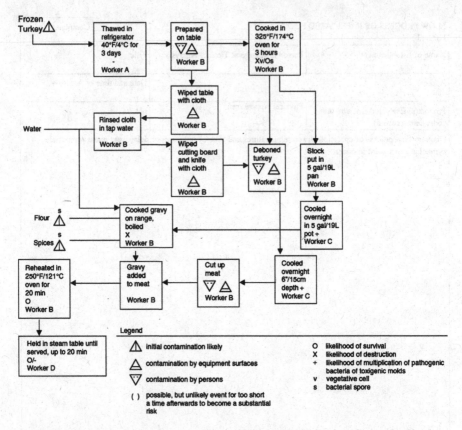

Fig. 10.3 Example completed form (see Fig. 10.2) likely used by local public health officials to investigate a foodborne illness claim and/or outbreak in a retail food service establishment. Reprinted with permission from Procedures to Investigate Foodborne Illness (Sixth Edition—2011). (Copyright held by the International Association for Food Protection, Des Moines, Iowa, USA. Available for purchase at http://www.foodprotection.org)

Having intimate knowledge of your HACCP plan and how procedures are supposed to be followed for each food prep procedure (and data to verify this) will be important to enable the public health official to rule in or rule out the implicated food by inspection of the facilities and observation of employee behaviors in the retail unit. If the HACCP plans are followed carefully in the retail unit (education evident and systems are validated), and the documented procedures can be verified during the investigation, it will enable the public health officials to quickly determine if the retail unit is associated with the foodborne outbreak or not. This can protect the business from being unintentionally associated with an outbreak, but just as importantly reduce cost and time to public health officials who may be investigating multiple retail facilities and/or manufacturing facilities to determine the source of the outbreak. Many foodborne illness investigations can more quickly implicate manufactured ingredients/products contaminated at the manufactures facility (as opposed to contaminated foods at retail), when a food retail unit can show record of proper receipt, preperation, and service of these effected foods; investigators gain more insight into the likely source of an outbreak using epidemiological methods of deduction.

Have Knowledge of How Outbreak Investigations Are Performed

There are two very helpful resources to learn more about how a foodborne disease outbreak investigation is performed. The first is the International Association for Food Protections manual, Procedures to Investigate Foodborne Illness (IAFP 2011). Although this manual was written by and for public health officials as a training tool to harmonize investigations, it can be a useful resource for the food safety professional responsible for retail food safety management. The second written resource is called the Guidelines for Foodborne Disease Outbreak Response (CIFOR 2009) produced by the council to improve foodborne disease outbreak response (CIFOR). These guidelines were written specifically for both industry and public health officials and were produced by several workgroups (made up of local, state, and federal partners including an industry workgroup). The industry workgroup was formed to foster partnerships between food safety professionals in public health and the food industry in order to improve foodborne outbreak detection and response. This resource can also be helpful in designing systems to improve foodborne illness claim surveillance, reporting, traceback, and recalls within a food retail business.

There are also two good resources of "hands on" training to gain more knowledge of how public health officials investigate foodborne disease illnesses and outbreaks. The first one has had significant industry input (via collaboration) called Industry-Foodborne Illness Investigation Training (I-FIIT, see NEHA 2012a). This training program was developed through a partnership between public health officials, industry, and NEHA. According to the NEHA, I-FIIT is a 1-day face-to-face workshop that both food service representatives and their appropriate local and state regulatory officials participate together in (at same training event) to create stronger working relationships prior to a potential foodborne disease incident occurring. The I-FIIT workshop also provides clarity on the investigation process by identifying the roles and responsibilities of industry and public health officials, teaching early detection strategies, and how to establish and implement hazard control measures based on model practices. I-FIIT's mission is to assist industry and regulatory officials to more quickly and effectively respond to foodborne illness incidents to reduce the number of cases of illness and death during a foodborne disease outbreak.

The second training program is a more advanced training on foodborne disease outbreak investigations called Epi-Ready Team Training: Foodborne Illness Response Strategies, and is also offered by the National Environmental Health Association (NEHA 2012a, b) co-developed with the CDC. This course is a more advanced training for food safety professionals (those with advanced degrees in public health or food science that work in local/state epidemiology and/or health departments) but can be easily comprehended by the retail food safety professional on the food safety management team. Epi-Ready is also face-to-face team-based training workshop usually attended by public health officials that can help the food safety management team be prepared to be involved with and help public health officials during a foodborne illness outbreak investigation.

Retail Regulatory Rules and Interpretation

The FDA Food Code was first published in 1993 as a model for state and local agencies that regulate food service, vending, and retail food stores. The food code is a set of rules based on current science and methods known to prevent hazards during retail food production (e.g., potentially hazardous foods should be stored at temperatures above 135 °F or below 41 °F to prevent pathogen growth or bacterial toxin production in the food) and is updated in part through proposals by the nonprofit organization called the Conference for Food Protection (CFP). The CFP provides a forum, as their Web site states "for representative and equitable partnership among regulators, industry, academia, professional organizations and consumers to identify problems, formulate recommendations, and develop and implement practices that ensure food safety. New rapidly developing food technologies and marketing innovations challenge all groups involved in food production and monitoring to work together to enhance the quality of our food supply" (Conference for Food Protection 2012). The CFP's primary channels for dissemination of information (to be considered for possible regulatory rule making) are the USDA/FSIS and the FDA.

Food safety professionals in the retail food business can participate on most councils, committees, and the executive board and can also serve as chair and vice-chair on most councils. Food safety professionals from industry are elected through industry caucuses, and the food industry's concerns and advice are fully considered in this forum. The food safety management team member can apply for membership to the CFP, request service on its councils as a means to build relationships with public health officials (among many state representatives), and partner to influence more operationally feasible rules (and cost-effective methods industry can meet) to better control hazards in retail food service establishments. Many times the knowledge gained through participation in the CFP (as well as other forums discussed below) can be used to develop improved SOPs within the retail food business before any regulatory requirement is developed and implemented.

Most states adopt the FDA Food Code with minor changes and thus measure and enforce these same rules in retail food service establishments within their state (see FDA 2011). However, not all states' rules are updated to the most current FDA Food Code (17% of these still base their state rules on pre-2001 FDA Food Codes, see Fig. 10.4). However, even though many states do not enforce the most current FDA rules, as discussed in Chap. 4 (Systems), it is best to base all corporate-directed retail procedures and training programs on the most current FDA Food Code rules to ensure both food safety and regulatory compliance in all states.

Some local jurisdictions have different food code rules than their state as well. Because, local regulatory public health officials, not the FDA, enforce the food code

State Food Code Adoptions

Forty-nine (49) of the 50 States adopted codes patterned after the 1993, 1995, 1997, 1999, 2001, 2005, or 2009 versions of the Food Code. These represent 96% of the US population. A breakdown by Food Code version follows:

- **Four** States adopted the 1993, 1995 or 1997 Food Code, representing 4% of the US population.

- **Ten** States adopted the 1999 Food Code, representing **13%** of the US population.

- **Eleven** States adopted the 2001 Food Code, representing **38%** of the US population.

- **Twenty one** States adopted the 2005 Food Code, representing **39%** of the US population.

- **Three** State adopted the 2009 Food Code, representing **2%** of the US population.

Fig. 10.4 Percent of states that have adopted the FDA Food Code and version of food code adopted (FDA 2011)

rules in each state, it is important to clearly understand each states (and local jurisdictions if applicable) specific food code rules (or minimally, the state you do retail business in). Therefore, an additional opportunity, and important partnership with public health officials, is to actively participate in a states food safety and defense task force. Many of these task force organizations are funded by the FDA to foster industry and government partnerships, and each can be easily located for membership application by searching the internet for "food safety and defense task force." Both Georgia and North Carolina, two i have experience with, support industry participation in their food safety and defense task force, and members have the chance to meet and discuss best practices to work together to reduce food safety hazards within the food industry.

Another area of importance to building partnerships is the knowledge of and participation with food code rules interpretation and how the state or local jurisdiction interprets these rules (i.e., how they expect the food retail unit to demonstrate compliance). Many states have developed an Interpretations Manual (see Georgia 2011) to aid in the training of their health inspectors on retail food code inspections, and it is important that the food safety management professional (and retail unit operators) understands these interpretations to be prepared for inspections and demonstrate compliance. For example, PART-I—"Administrative Guidance to Interpretation of the Georgia Food Service Rules and Regulations Chapter 290-5-14"—has two parts that empower a food retail business to inquire about how the state interprets/enforces application of a rule (Section A below) and gain guidance for interpretation (Section B).

Section A—Interpretations: Provides for the administrative procedures for the submittal of interpretative request regarding the application of the Chapter's Food Service Rules and Regulations. It also establishes the administrative procedures for responding to interpretative requests received by the Division.

Section B—Public Health Reasons and Administrative Guidelines: Provides for the public health reasons and administrative guidance for the interpretation of Georgia's Food Service Rules and Regulations Chapter 290-5-14. Section B does not address all of the Rules and Regulations within Chapter 290-5-14. However, it does address the most frequent inquiries of specific Rules and Regulations received by the Division since the adoption of the Chapter by the Department in February of 2007.

Clearly it is important to know how regulatory officials (e.g., health inspectors) interpret rules applied during inspections if the retail food business is to ensure compliance of its procedures and achieve positive inspection scores/grades. More importantly, when interpretations are unclear, this partnership can support understanding and variance to a rule as long as the interpretation (e.g., alternative procedure) meets the requirements/reasons for the rule to ensure food safety.

Food Safety Forums

Another area of partnership where the food safety management team can interact with public health officials and work together in the mission to prevent foodborne illness is in participation with industry and government forums. Food safety professionals meet at many of these national and international forums organized by industry trade groups (e.g., National Restaurant Association, International Association for Food Protection, Global Food Safety Initiative, Institute of Food Technologists, Food Marketing Institute, National Environmental Health Association, and Association of Food and Drug Officials). Many of these organizations host poster sessions on the latest academic and industry supported research on food safety improvements and offer expos where businesses involved in the sale of food safety solutions (tools, chemical, and services) demonstrate their products.

Benefits Beyond Public Health

There are additional business benefits to partnering with public health officials. These benefits to partnership include:

- Provide valuable resources, tools, and subject matter experts to give council on food safety management program work
- Key contacts for sources of information during local and national foodborne diseases outbreak investigations (to be prepared for possible actions needed to protect the business)
- Key contacts in states where natural disasters may affect retail business operations
- Knowledge of how to submit variance request of food code rule interpretations to ensure compliance

The food retail business is in the business of food safety because it must sell safe food to stay in business and oftentimes show public health officials evidence of this. Partnering with public health officials is therefore good business.

References

Barton Behravesh C et al (2011) 2008 outbreak of Salmonella Saintpaul infections associated with raw produce. N Engl J Med 364:918–927

CDC (2012) CDC estimates of foodborne illness in the United States. Available via internet at http://www.cdc.gov/foodborneburden/2011-foodborne-estimates.html/

CIFOR (2009) Guidelines for foodborne disease outbreak response. Available via internet at http://www.cifor.us/toolkit.cfm

Conference for Food Protection (2012) Available via internet at http://www.foodprotect.org/

FDA News Release (2008a) FDA warns consumers nationwide not to eat certain types of raw red tomatoes. Available via internet at http://www.fda.gov/NewsEvents/Newsroom/PressAnnouncements/2008/ucm116908.htm

FDA News Release (2008b) FDA lifts warning about eating certain types of tomatoes. Available via internet at http://www.fda.gov/NewsEvents/Newsroom/PressAnnouncements/2008/ucm116923.htm

FDA (2011) Real progress in food code adoptions. Available via internet at http://www.fda.gov/Food/FoodSafety/RetailFoodProtection/FederalStateCooperativePrograms/ucm108156.htm

Georgia (2011) Food service interpretation manual. Available via internet at http://health.state.ga.us/programs/envservices/FSManual.asp

IAFP (2011) Procedures to investigate foodborne illness, 6th edn. Springer, Heidelberg

Meyerson A (2009) An analysis of the first-order economic costs of the 2008 FDA tomato warning. Available via internet at http://web-docs.stern.nyu.edu/glucksman/docs/Meyerson2009.pdf

NEHA (2012a) Epi-Ready team training: foodborne illness response strategies. Available via internet at http://www.neha.org/epi_ready/index.html

NEHA (2012b) Industry: foodborne illness investigation training (I-FIIT). Available via internet at http://www.neha.org/ifiit/index.html

Index